GW00721780

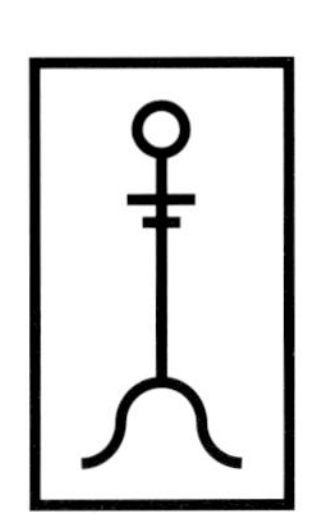

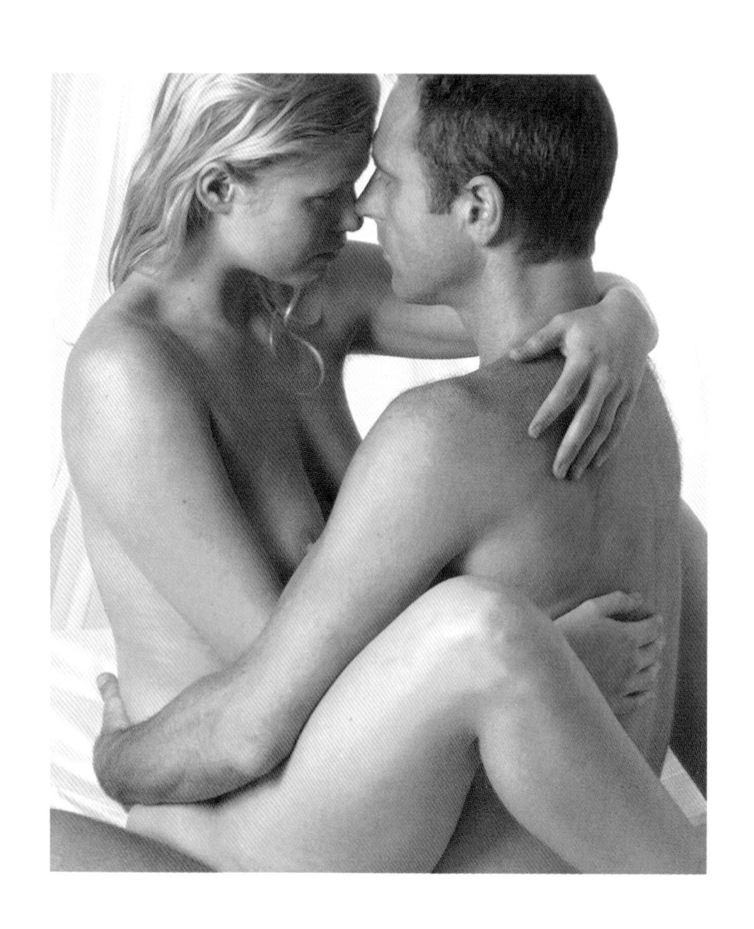

ECSTATIC SEX

A Guide to the Pleasures of Tantra

MA ANANDA SARITA *and* SWAMI ANAND GEHO

A Fireside Book

Published by Simon & Schuster

New York London Toronto Sydney Singapore

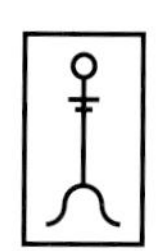

FIRESIDE
Rockefeller Center
1230 Avenue of the Americas
New York, NY 10020

For information regarding special discounts for bulk purchases,please contact
Simon & Schuster Special Sales at 1-800-456-6798 or business@simonandschuster.com

Designed by Lucy Guenot

Printed in Singapore by Imago

10 9 8 7 6 5 4 3 2 1

Library of Congress Cataloging-in-Publication Data

Sarita, Ma Ananda.

Ecstatic sex : a guide to the pleasures of Tantra / Ma Ananda Sarita and Swami Anand Geho.

p. cm.

ISBN 0-7432-4610-1 (alk.paper)

1. Sex instruction. 2. Sex. 3. Tantrism. I Geho, Swami Anand. II. Title.

HQ64.S34 2003

613.9'6-dc21

2003045568

PUBLISHER'S NOTE

The meditations, ideas, and suggestions in this book are to be used at the reader's sole discretion and risk. Always follow the instructions closely, and consult a doctor if you are worried about a physical or psychological problem.

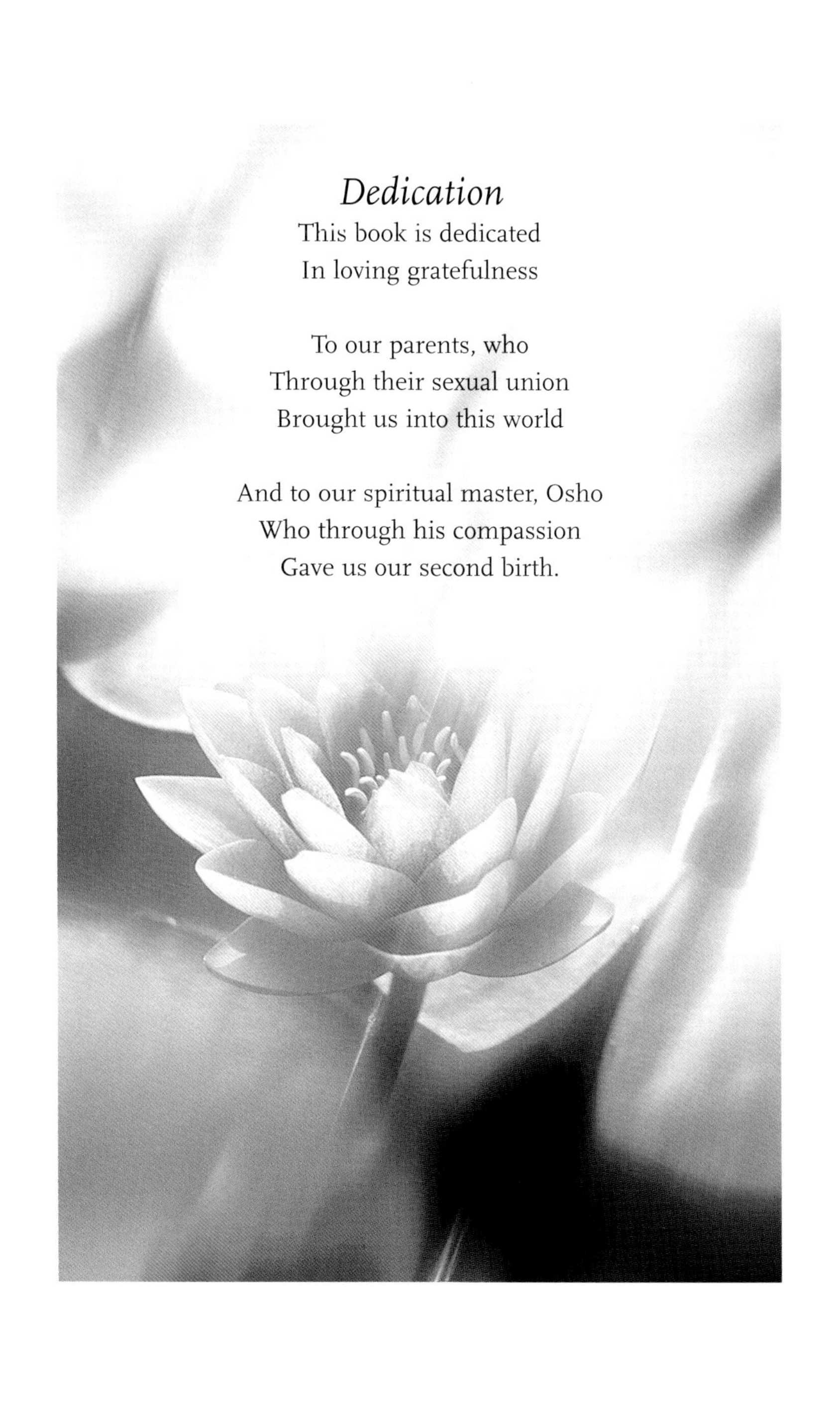

Dedication

This book is dedicated
In loving gratefulness

To our parents, who
Through their sexual union
Brought us into this world

And to our spiritual master, Osho
Who through his compassion
Gave us our second birth.

contents

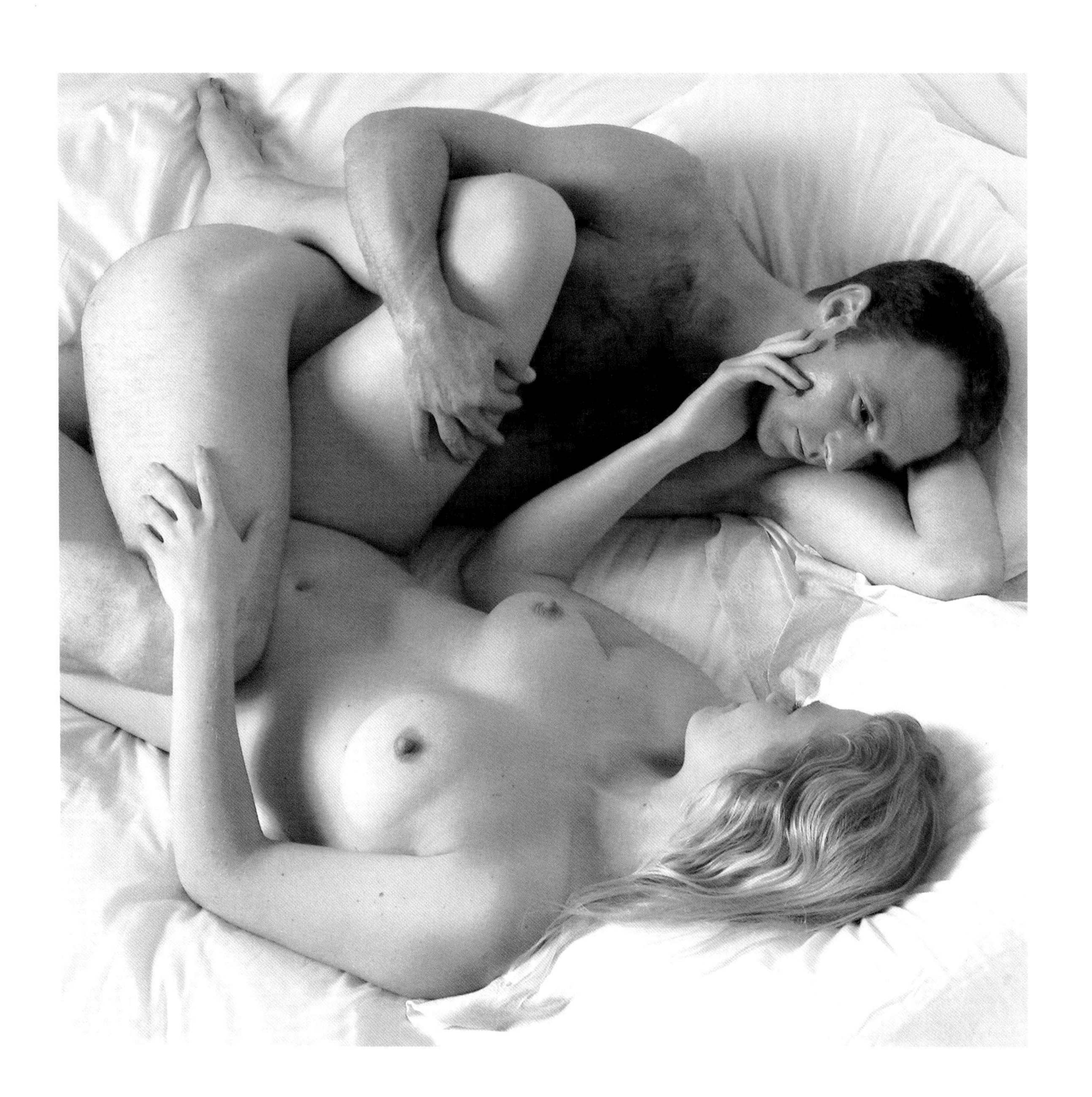

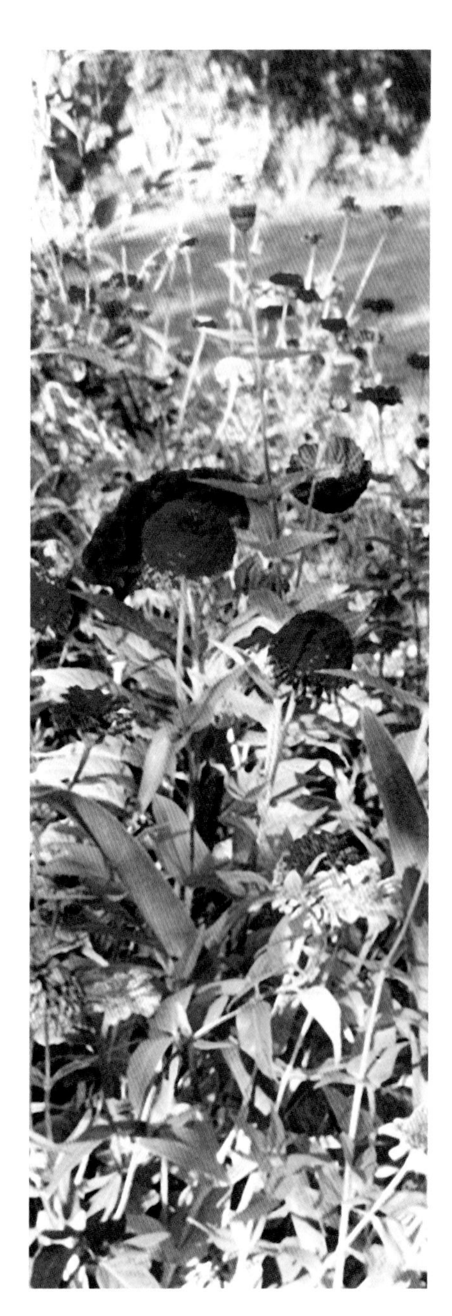

introduction

This book is borne to you on the wings of our experience as a Tantric couple. We both arrived in India at the age of 17, searching for the essence of life. At that time we didn't know one another, even though we were initiated by the same Master, Osho into the mysteries of Tantra as a meditative path to spiritual liberation. Sarita remained in India for 26 years, and Geho for 20 years. During that time, we were each exploring all the facets of our being, moving closer and closer to our true natures. This path has been described like moving on a razor's edge, because to combine meditation with love and sex, as practiced in Tantra, needs a heightened degree of sensitivity and awareness. In the community around our Master, we had the freedom to explore every facet of our sexuality and were thus challenged to discover sex as a doorway to heightened consciousness.

Those looking at Tantra from the outside can misunderstand this path, and due to such misunderstanding our Master was dubbed the "Sex Guru" by the press. However, his radical methods for transforming human consciousness attracted thousands of people, from many nations and all walks of life, giving rise to concern among some people that this movement could bring about an earthquake of change in the collective psyche of society. His teaching is simply the subjective path of self-transformation, from sex to superconsciousness.

Having absorbed his teaching and been transformed through it, when Osho left his body in 1990 we were ready to begin sharing what we had learned. Initially both of us chose holistic healing arts as an avenue of expression. Geho became a massage therapist and teacher and Sarita became a Color Light Therapist and teacher. It was during our work in the healing arts that we met and became friends, in the early 1990s.

In 1994 we decided to embark on an experiment. We both wished to explore deeply, and yet in a scientific way, the effect of a series of Tantra meditations to be practiced in sex. We scheduled 28 Tantra meditation appointments, with the agreement that no matter what arose emotionally, mentally, or physically, we would see the appointments through to their conclusion. After that, we would be free of any commitment. Each appointment took place in a sacred space we had consecrated for the occasion. We began by invoking higher consciousness to bless our union. We bowed down to the principle of love itself, as embodied in each other. And during the meditation, we kept uppermost the remembrance that this man and this woman represented the feminine principle and the masculine principle, beyond personality. We regarded each other as god and goddess. In this setting, and through our Tantra practice together, we were both transformed beyond what we had ever dreamed was possible between a man and a woman. Our sexual experience was lifted up into the purifying fire of love. We discovered, as it is said in Tantra, that sex and Samadhi (spiritual awakening) are one.

After this experience, we returned to our ordinary everyday reality, letting go of all Tantra meditation practice and giving time for the transformation to be integrated. We discovered that this is a valuable approach, allowing the pendulum to swing in both directions. The first series of meditations were so powerful in their effect, that after some time we decided to embark on another series. We continued in this way, scheduling series of Tantra appointments, and then letting go into ordinariness, back and forth, back and forth, giving equal space to both dimensions. One day, by surprise, while we were in our ordinary phase, the pendulum arrived in the middle. Our godly and human aspects met in deep union. This experience brought with it a sudden awakening and a deep crystallization of our inner mastery of Tantra. The Tantra path became so clear to us that we found ourselves very naturally inspired to share our discovery through Tantra groups. We devised a seven-level Tantra training for couples and a three-level Tantra training for singles. Subsequently we moved to Europe, where our teaching was received with gratefulness and enthusiasm.

During our years of teaching, working with couples and individuals from many different nationalities, of all ages and from a variety of backgrounds, we have discovered that sharing the Tantric way of life is really all about helping people to

The Tantric way of life is really all about helping people to remember and embrace what is already inside. Each person carries both human and divine qualities. Each person carries sexuality, animality, and sacredness as an integral part of their being. The art and science of Tantra is really all about helping these opposite qualities to meet and merge, giving birth to an alchemical refinement of being, where sex and spirituality can be celebrated as an integrated whole.

remember and embrace what is already inside. Each person carries both human and divine qualities; sexuality, animality, and sacredness are an integral part of our being. The art and science of Tantra is helping these opposite qualities to meet and merge, giving birth to a refinement of being, where sex and spirituality can be celebrated as an integrated whole.

We wrote a book, *Tantric Love*, focusing on the meditative and spiritual aspects of a Tantric love union. The book is a rich reminder of what we are all capable of discovering through the dedicated practice of Tantra methods. After writing it, we realized that a second book was waiting to be born – and this is the one you now hold in your hands. It has been written in response to the thirst people have to discover a balanced, uplifting sexual expression, freed from puritanical ideas, without getting lost in a quagmire of licentiousness. We have found that many people of all ages have been groping in the dark with this most basic human need, and suffering as a result. As people grow up there seem to be no guidelines for a refined and ecstatic sexuality. It is not taught in a satisfying way, and this seems to be because our society as a whole is quite lost and confused around sex and sexual relating. One woman of 84 said to us, "I know Tantra is my next step. In fact, it has always been a part of me. But when I was growing up there was simply no information about it available. I had no choice but to take on board the repressive attitudes of society. Now, I fear it may be too late for me." This courageous woman, after our conversation, was able to manifest a Tantra partner in her life. Her story (see chapter 21) is a poignant reminder that it is never too late to begin a fulfilling, nurturing Tantra relationship.

This book is for people of all ages and from all walks of life. No matter what our differences of race, age, or creed, we were all born out of sex. Sexual arousal, and subsequent courtship, gives rise to both rapture and pain. Great poetry, sculpture, dance, music, painting, and drama are woven around our human need to explore deep sexual love. Understanding its secrets can positively transform human relationships and our approach toward society. Sex is such a powerful force that it may throw us into the deepest despair if practiced in ignorance. Conversely, it can bring us to the most sublime states of bliss and understanding if practiced with intelligence. Therefore it makes sense to shine the light of our most refined intelligence on this fascinating subject.

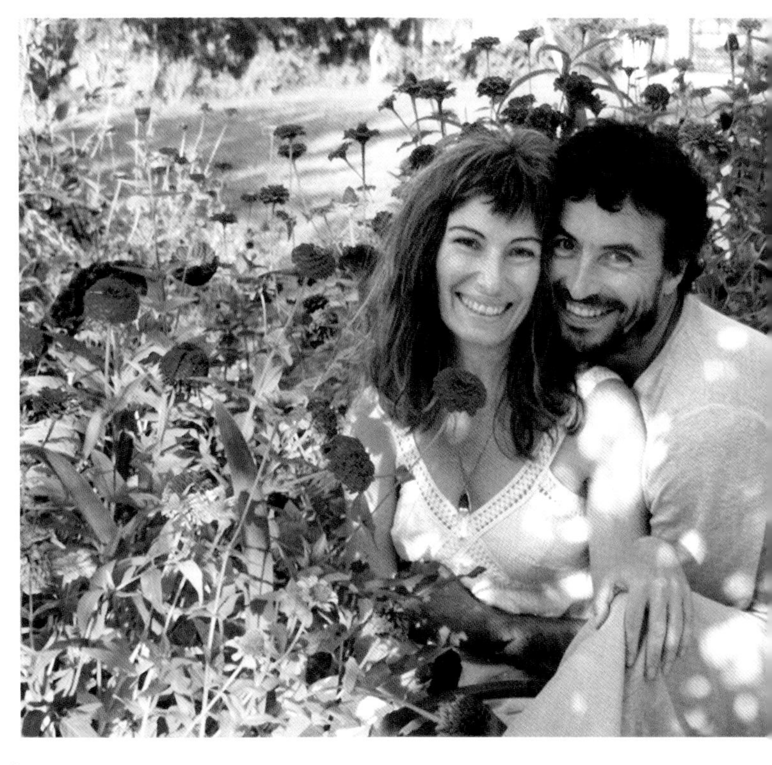

We offer here our research and insights into Tantric sex, knowing that these may be but a drop in the ocean of the vast potential of human understanding around this subject. We have endeavoured to address the invisible barriers and taboos that keep people cut off from their potential for ecstatic sex. With this in mind, we provide very basic information (everything you wanted to know about sex but were too shy to ask) as well as providing exercises and methods to help you explore your sexual potential from the balanced perspective of Tantra. We have also gone deeply into the difference between men and women and how this difference can become a harmony of opposites.

It is our belief that human happiness born out of fulfilled sensuality is the cornerstone of a balanced society. Through this book we hope to contribute to a positive transformation of our society. If we, who grew up as normally conditioned and sexually ignorant members of Western culture, could discover the ecstatic transformation offered by Tantra, then such transformation is certainly possible for anyone willing to devote themselves to it.

We wish you blessings and love in your continuing discovery of what it means to become an ecstatic human being.

With love,

Geho Sarita

Geho and Sarita

France, January 2003

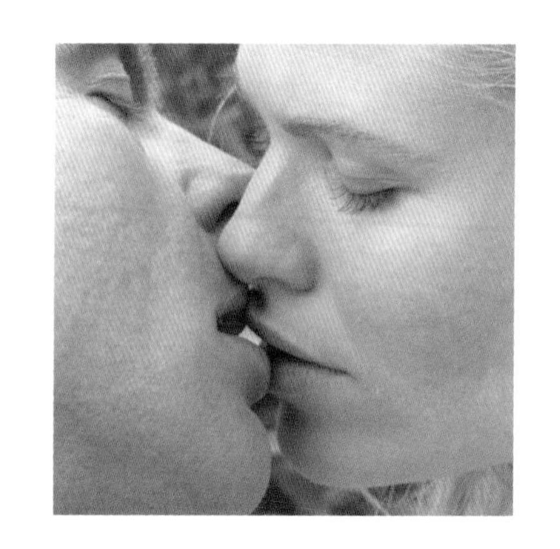

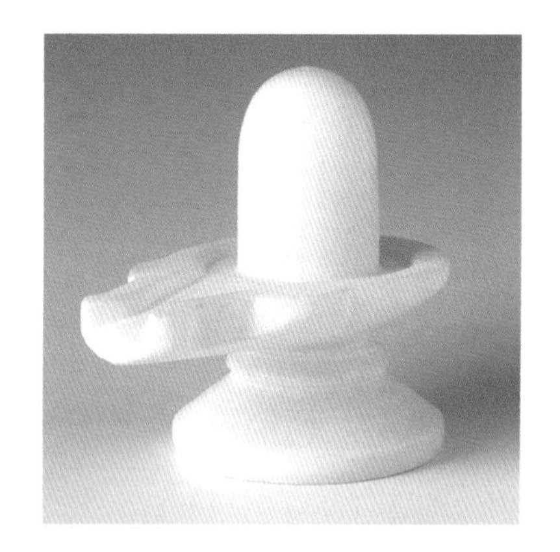

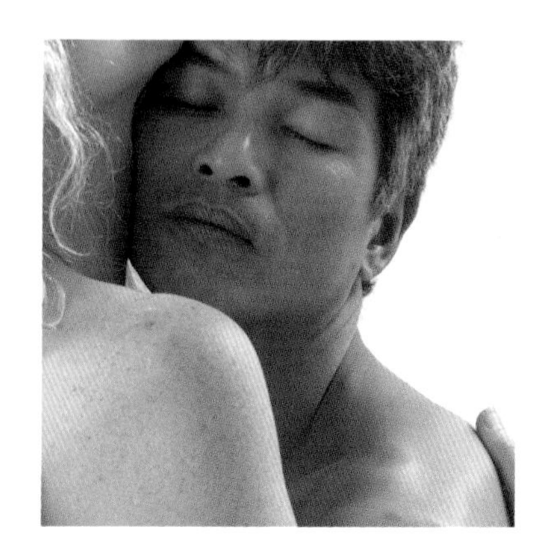

part 1

the body

The body is a microcosm of the macrocosm, a universe of discovery. Learning about and tapping into the intelligent network of communication that forms the body/mind is an important step in understanding and enhancing sexual relations. This adventure of discovery begins with love and appreciation for your own body. Knowing your body as worthy of respect helps your sexual pleasure to flower.

In Tantra we use Sanskrit names for the genitals, since these carry a profound message for enhancing pleasure even further. Lingam (the male genitals) means "pillar of light"; Yoni (the female genitals) means "sacred place". By transforming everyday sexuality into sacred sexuality, you lift the experience of sex into its refined aspect; it is a door leading to superconsciousness. Thus a knowledge of the anatomy of the Lingam and Yoni broadens your understanding, empowering you to embrace your full ecstatic potential. The dynamism of these male and female qualities uniting has profound implications for human health and happiness.

chapter 1

your body is sacred

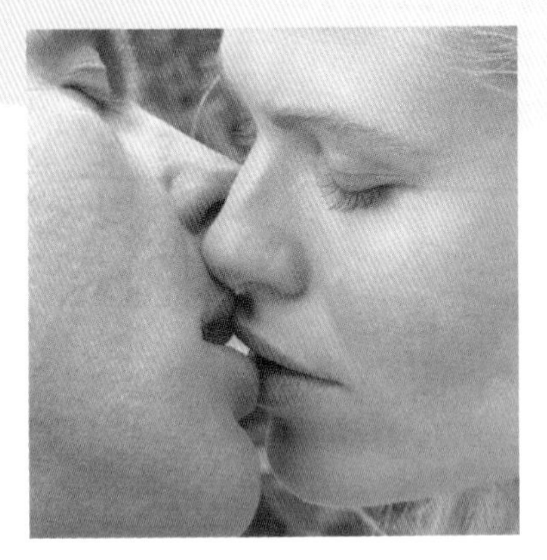

"My Dove, in the cliffs of the rocks, the secret of steep ravines
Come let me look at you, come let me hear you
Your voice clear as water, your beautiful body"
From the Bible, *The Song of Songs*, translated by Marcia Falk

Your body is a miracle. There are millions of cells in the human body, all working together moment by moment like musicians in an orchestra, in eloquent and harmonious communication. It is through our bodies that we experience all the pleasures life can bring – all the sensory experiences, including taste, smell, sight, emotion, orgasm, and ecstasy.

In fact, to talk about the "body" is inaccurate, since the body and mind are one integrated networking system. What you think or feel emotionally affects your body, and how you experience your physical energy affects your mind. We often think that the body is simply a mechanism, but really it is an extension of the brain and carries a highly refined quality of intelligence. Whether you are awake or sleeping, it goes on functioning in the best possible way without much awareness on your part.

Because the body functions so smoothly, you may give it little thought unless you feel pain or sickness. But your happiness and enjoyment of life depend on your bodily wellbeing. Health and happiness go together – it is very difficult to experience much pleasure or love if you are ill, in pain, or just not feeling your best. Candace Pert, a scientist who has made breakthrough discoveries on the body/mind connection says: "I believe that happiness is what we feel when our biochemicals of emotion, the neuropeptides and their receptors are open and flowing freely throughout the psychosomatic network, integrating and co-ordinating our systems, organs and cells in a smooth and rhythmic movement. ... I believe that happiness is our natural state, that bliss is hardwired."

Your thoughts, your emotions, what you eat and drink, and your living environment, all affect the functioning of your body. All these elements enter into the communication stream, where incoming information is passed on to every body cell.

As conscious human beings, we have free will. We are only partially programmed by instinct. A large part of our body/mind is programmed through our physical and psychological environment. This brings tremendous freedom, making us adaptable to all kinds of conditions. But it also brings great responsibility. Through the environment we choose, we are simultaneously programming our physical and mental functioning.

This is the basis for Feng Shui, which creates positive changes in all aspects of life by bringing harmony to architecture and interior design. Certain approaches to food, including Ayurveda, macrobiotics, and instinctotherapy, help to nourish health, emotional stability, and a sense of happiness. The need for loving touch is something we never grow out of. Touch, or lack of it, is also a crucial environmental factor.

Mental stimulus is another important aspect. Your mind is a "bio-computer", easily programmed by what it is subjected to. For example, if you watch violence on television you are installing a tendency toward violence in your brain. However, if you nurture your brain with exquisite music or scenes of beauty, you are refining your mental capacity. Your mind will respond by opening toward sensitivity, creativity, and love.

The more you give yourself an inner and outer environment of nurturing and love, the more you will encourage the fullest flowering of what you can be: vibrant, ecstatic, and wise.

Loving yourself is a far stronger force than will-power – more women should try it. I stopped eating cakes and fries and burgers because I believed my body deserved much better. Now the whole idea of putting a cream cake into my system is just gross. Why would I want to clog myself up with all that fat?

Jennifer Lopez, singer and actress

Self-love

Your fullest potential becomes activated as you learn to love yourself. Self-love starts with the body and is the beginning of all other kinds of love. If you cannot love yourself, how can you love and be loved by others? A person who hates their own body radiates that energy in their aura, and will therefore appear repulsive to others. A person who loves their body radiates such delight that they are magnetically attractive to others.

Many people complain that true love has not happened to them or to their relationships. The fact is that they do not love and care for their body/mind, but rather use it more like a garbage dump for unexpressed emotions, junk food, and low quality or violent mental stimulus. Discovering awe of the body/mind and living in vibrant body awareness will lead very naturally to nourishing relationships with others and a fulfilled sexuality. Fulfilling sexuality is simply an overflowing of pleasure born out of your total life energy. Nourish and love your whole being and your sexual expression will mirror it.

Very few people are encouraged to appreciate and care for their body as they grow up. Loving your body is something you have to discover as a kind of self-education. The food you eat and drink, the way you look at yourself in the mirror, the way you touch your body, the way you think or talk about yourself, the care you give your body – all that is your responsibility; others can't do it for you. When you love and respect yourself, not judging your outward appearance, you create such an aura of love and caring around yourself that both you and others benefit from it, and start responding to it with more love. Fashion surveys have found that the clothes you wear are not what make an impression on others. It is how you feel about yourself that creates a lasting impression on the people you meet. Your clothes are only a reflection of how you feel inside. That is how you create your own reality: what you think and live inside and what you express go on resounding around yourself and come back to you, reflected by others and ultimately the whole of existence.

Loving your body is something you have to discover as a kind of self-education. The food you eat and drink, the way you look at yourself in the mirror, the way you touch your body, the way you think or talk about yourself, the care you give your body – all that is your responsibility; others can't do it for you.

One of the wonderful teachings of Tantra is that the body is the sacred temple, the abode of the divine. We can evolve with the body to expand our consciousness and reach higher levels of bliss. Tantra has developed methods and meditations using very diverse bodily experiences such as breathing, dancing, singing, sipping tea, touching, making love, and orgasm. Any bodily experiences can catapult us into an expanded state of being, where body, mind, and soul function as one harmonious whole. Creating this state of harmony always begins with appreciation and care of your own body.

The ultimate potential of the body is to create a place where love, bliss, and the highest peak of human consciousness, an orgasmic oneness with the whole of life known as Mahamudra, can happen.

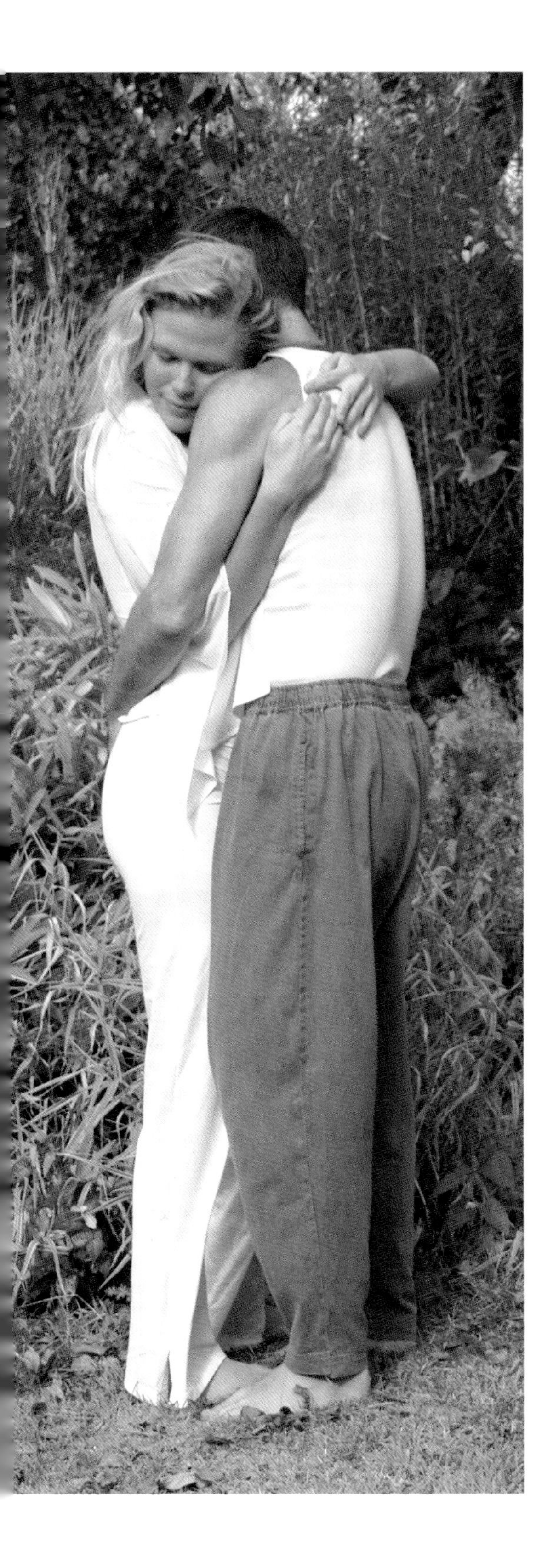

tips to enhance body love

♡ Eat healthy and fresh foods, preferably organically grown.
Drink pure, high-quality water.
Give yourself the gift of a nourishing and balanced diet.

♡ Take regular exercise such as walking, dancing, swimming, or playful non-competitive sports.

♡ Receive full-body massage regularly, ideally once a week.

♡ Embrace friends or your lover daily
(we never grow out of the need to cuddle).

♡ Enter into sex play on a regular basis,
either with a willing partner or with yourself.

♡ When you see your naked body in the mirror, look with the eyes of someone in love. Keep searching for new aspects of your body to appreciate.

♡ Remember, beauty arises from how you experience yourself from within.

How fine
You are my love
Your eyes like doves
Behind your veil

Your hair –
As black as goats
Winding down the slopes

Your teeth –
A flock of sheep
Rising from the stream
In twos, each with its twin

Your lips –
Like woven threads
Of crimson silk

A gleam of pomegranate –
Your forehead
Through your veil

Your neck –
A tower
Adorned with shields

Your breasts –
Twin fauns
In fields of flowers

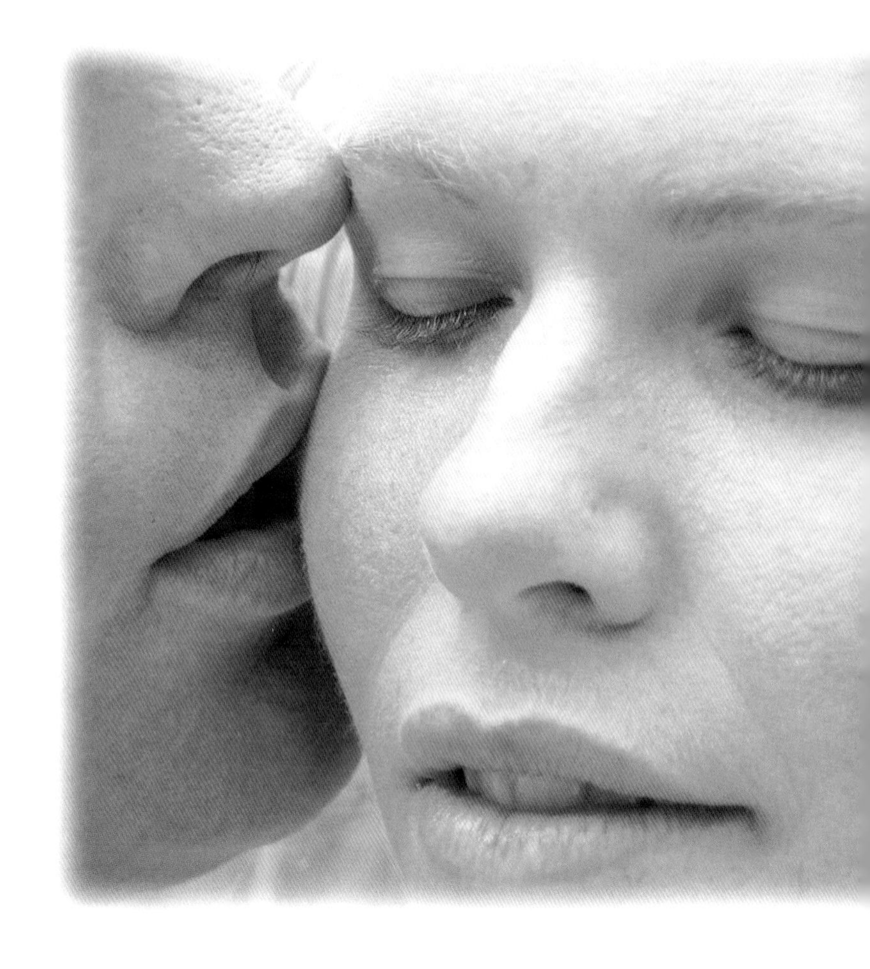

from *The Song of Songs,* translated by Marcia Falk

a date with yourself

Try this truly liberating experience.

Make a date with yourself. For the whole day, look forward to it with great anticipation – the hot date you have always dreamed of.

Bathe luxuriously and dress up in something that you feel really special in. Tell yourself out loud how amazing you look and what a gift it is to have this special time with yourself.

Go out wining and dining in an ambience that really touches you with pleasure. Take yourself to a dance or to an opera, or wherever you will enjoy an uplifting experience.

During the whole evening, whisper soft endearments to yourself and allow that magic glow of someone very much in love to fill you.

Take yourself home for a night-cap and perhaps a slow romantic dance, hugging yourself.

Then take yourself to bed and undress yourself slowly, marvelling at how amazing you are, how beautiful, how divinely sexy.

Make love to yourself, holding nothing back. You are the best lover in the world. You are the one you have been waiting for.

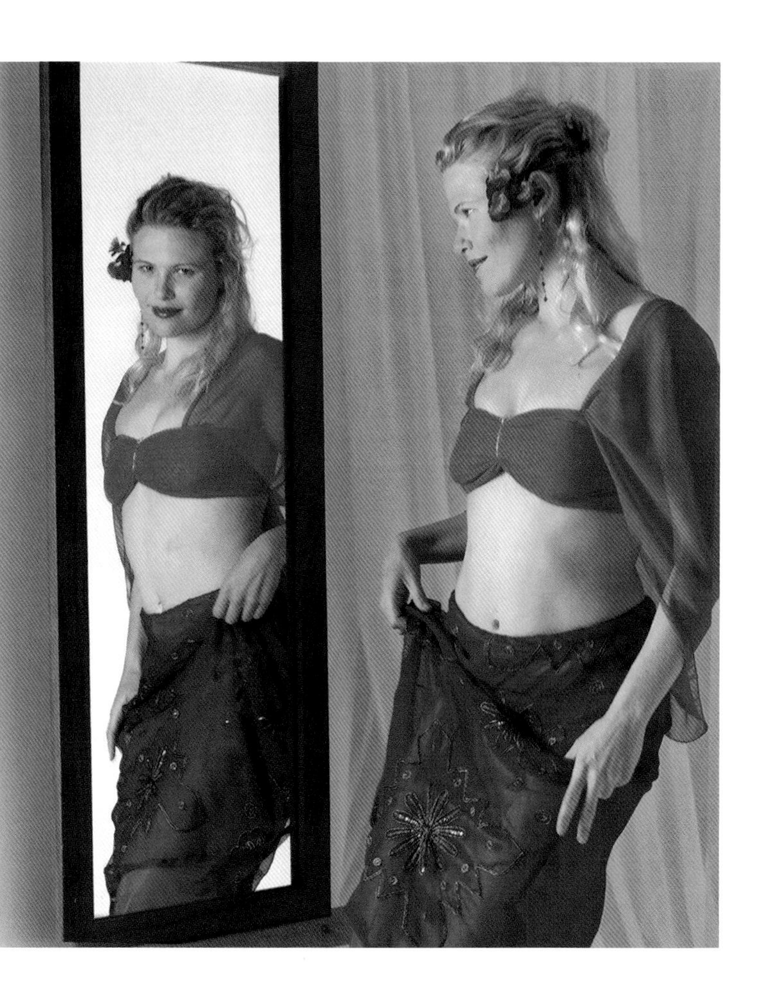

Make a date with yourself a few times. The experience is life-transforming, because once you are in love with yourself, you become magnetically attractive to others. Your inner glow of fulfilment is irresistible.

chapter 2

Yoni and Lingam

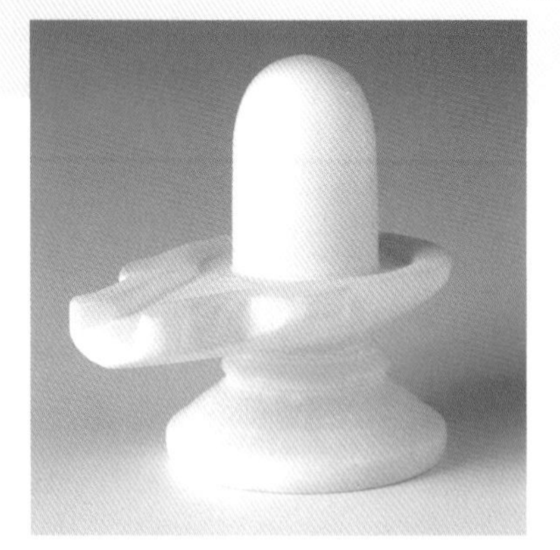

"Universal energy, the substance of the world, is represented by the yoni which grasps the lingam. It is only when the phallus, the giver of semen, is surrounded by the yoni that God can manifest and the universe appear."
Karpatri, Sanskrit scripture, translated by Alain Danielou

The Yoni

Each woman is a goddess because each Yoni is the custodian of the infinite mystery of existence. Yoni is the Sanskrit word for the entire female genital system. It is softer than the English word, vagina, and far more poetic than the crude terms used in common speech. The Yoni is a sacred place.

Tantra is a life approach, born in India at a time when women were revered as incarnations of the great mother goddess. The Yoni is a symbol of the universal womb, from which all creation emerges and into which it dissolves back.

In Tantra, a male student will sit in front of his consort and meditate on her Yoni. If the male Tantrica does not have a physical Yoni to meditate on, he can meditate instead on a downward-pointing triangle with a black dot in the center. This dot, known as a Bindu, represents simultaneously the void from which springs creation, the divine mother, and the Yoni. This contemplation gives rise to an inner wisdom about the nature of the cosmos, because the woman's Yoni is a microcosm of the macrocosm from which all creation emerges.

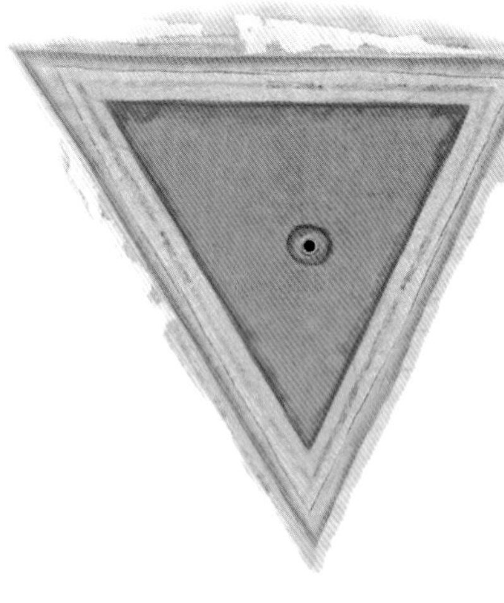

"Concentrate on the triangle of origination in the midst of space."

Hevajra Tantra

The power of Yoni worship

In many ancient cultures throughout the world, women were revered as birth-givers. The role of the male in conception was not always understood, and men were excluded and became jealous. Eventually they found that they could dominate the feminine, right-brained qualities through the development of left-brained advances in intellect, science, and technology. But there is a high price to pay for the tremendous technological advances that make our lives materially comfortable. Our mother earth is dying under the strain of the rapist technology, which devours natural resources and gives back only pollution. People suffer under the domination of greed-motivated governments, which have within them no balancing female qualities such as love and nurturing. In the past 30 years, we have destroyed one third of the world's natural resources. If we continue at the present rate, it is obvious what the future holds.

Reverence for the Yoni and for the feminine principle has tremendous implications for the world. Because the feminine principle is based on love, acceptance, and nurturing, Yoni worship can transform society. Tantra keeps this reverence in balance, by honouring the male and female principles equally. One sex does not need to dominate the other. Both can work together in co-operation, co-creation and interdependence, opposite and yet complementary poles of human existence.

Yoni worship is one of the oldest forms of religion and it continues today in many cultures of the world, including India, Japan, Aboriginal Australia, and South America. All our modern patriarchies are built on the foundation of Yoni-worshipping goddess-oriented religions. But the patriarchal attitude successfully smothered the reverence for the Yoni and the feminine, and continues to do so. Women still wear high heels (which raise the bottom into a provocative position, but damage the feet and lower back), a sign of their enslavement as a sex object – the modern equivalent of the ancient Chinese practice of foot-binding. Many women hate their Yonis, thinking that they look ugly and smell disgusting. Many women have no idea of when they are ovulating or of the mechanics of menstruation, pregnancy, and childbirth, blindly leaving all that in the hands of (mostly male) doctors. Many women live in anguish because they have not discovered the liberating power of their orgasmic being. Many women hate men because they feel they have been cheated by a dream of love, which has never come true.

In our society some women have tried to gain equality by copying men, but this only serves to disempower women. A woman's genitals clearly reveal that she is made opposite and yet complementary to man. This does not make her less than a man. When a woman discovers and accepts her own nature she will come into awareness of her unique power and beauty. This journey of acceptance and empowerment begins with her Yoni.

In Tantra texts the Yoni is the symbol of the creation principle. Worlds are both devoured by her and born out of her. She is the cosmic mother from where comes all life. And yet, her vengeful nature destroys all hope of clinging to life and her darkness is all pervading. These two faces she exhibits uphold the entire world. Know her and you have known all. Ignore her and you will be tormented, finding no peace. Love her and find the balm for your soul. Try to crush her and you will be lost to yourself, a wanderer in the desert of despair. Worship her and you will know peace and abundance within all the cycles of creation.

Each letter of the word Yoni has its own ineffable meaning in Sanskrit.

Y means the animating principle, the heart, the true self, union.

O means Preservation, brightness.

N means lotus, motherhood, menstrual cycle, nakedness, emptiness, pearl.

I means love, desire, consciousness, to shine, to pervade, pain and sorrow.

From *The Yoni*, by Rufus C Camphausen

The anatomy of the Yoni

Anatomically the clitoral crown is similar to the head of the penis, while the clitoral network, which is comprised of two cavernous bulbs on either side of the vulva, is in a sense like an introverted penis (or a penis is an extroverted vulva). Freud believed that women suffer from penis envy, but this whole idea is rather silly. In the foetus the male and female genitals are exactly the same until seven weeks' gestation, when hormonal changes cause them either to develop outside the body (male) or to remain and develop inside (female). Because so much of the Yoni is inside the body, people have imagined that there is less to it than there is to the male penis. In fact, in arousal the female genitals are equal in size to the male genitals and of a similar shape. The vagina acts as the bio-electric "socket" for the male "plug", giving rise to a deeply nurturing bio-electric current when they meet.

honoring your Yoni

In discovering and honoring your divine goddess nature embodied in your Yoni, you shower blessings on humanity. Through you, the goddess awakens and the balance of creation is renewed.

♡ If you think your Yoni smells bad, consider what you eat and avoid "junk" foods. The maxim "you are what you eat" applies directly to your Yoni. If you eat garlic, your Yoni will smell of it for three days. If you eat fresh vegetables and fruits, your Yoni will have a delightful fragrance. Drink pure water to help your body flush out toxins.

♡ Wash your Yoni inside and out with water, using gentle loving fingers. You should wash inside (without soap) daily during ovulation and menstruation and after each lovemaking session.

♡ Learn the language of female orgasm (see chapters 4 and 5). It is never too late to begin.

Gaze into a flower and marvel at its color, its intricate shape and design. The Yoni is more magnificent than all the flowers of the world.

Labia majora: outer lips of the female genitals, containing scent and sweat glands; they swell during arousal.

Labia minora: inner lips of the female genitals, usually hidden by the outer lips; they swell during arousal and secrete scent and moisture.

Clitoral crown: highly sensitive focal point for arousal and orgasm, containing approximately 3000 nerve endings devoted to pleasure. Normally hidden by the clitoral hood, during arousal it may swell and come out of hiding.
The venous erectile chambers form two separate arms from the clitoral crown. During arousal they become swollen and hypersensitive.

Hymen: a thin membrane of skin, covering the vaginal opening, broken by penetration or through exercise. (Not present in all girls or women.)

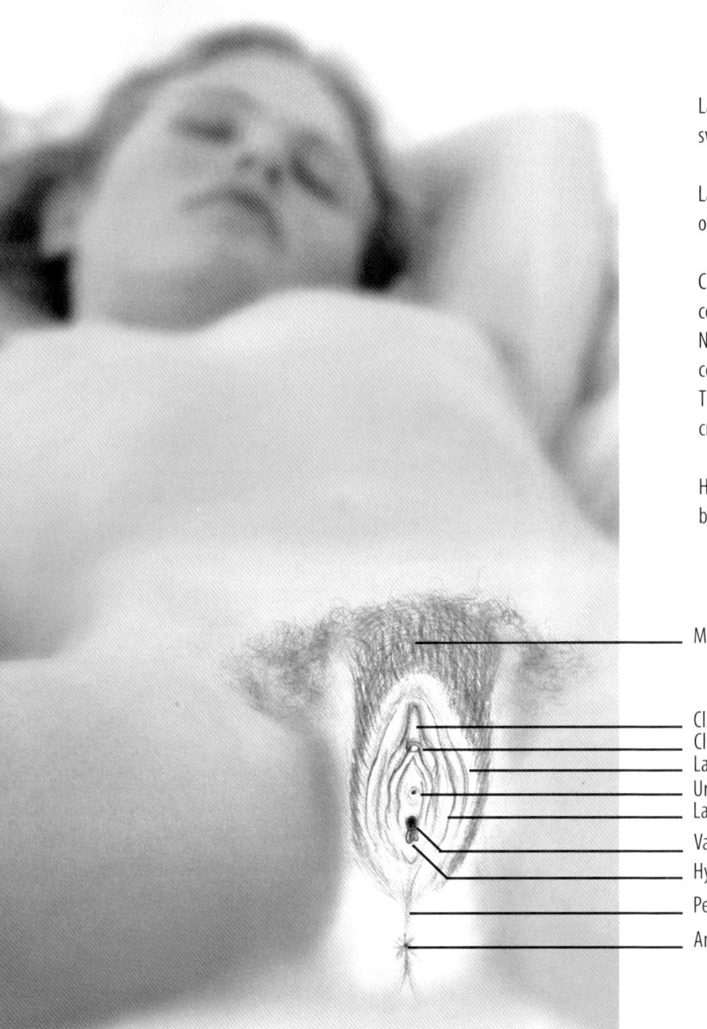

Fallopian tubes: allow the egg to travel from the ovaries to the womb; fertilization often takes place here.

Ovaries: where the eggs are stored; one egg ripens and is released each month.

Cervix: the opening of the womb

Urethral sponge or G-Spot (see page 51).

Bartholin's glands: either side of the vaginal opening; secrete an aphrodisiac scent and lubricating fluids.

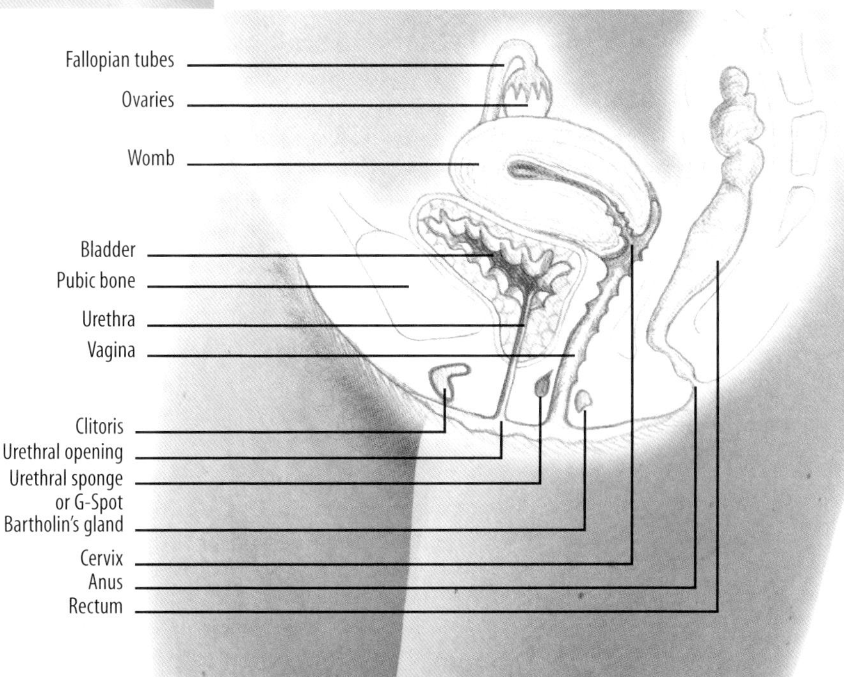

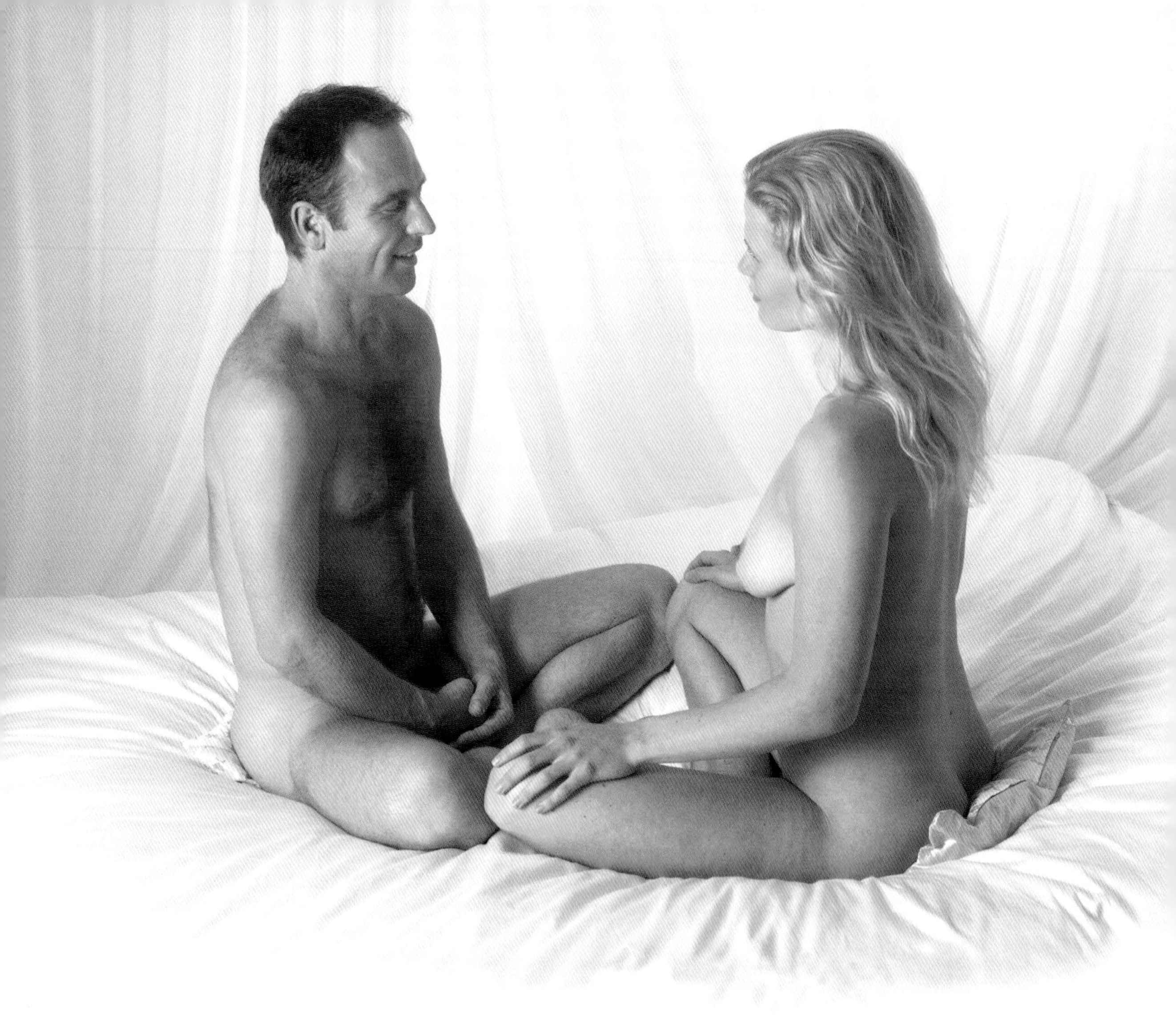

channelling Yoni and Lingam

This is an exercise for lovers to awaken, open, and reveal the many dimensions of the male and female genitals. It brings tremendous intimacy and is a good preparation for lovemaking. Practice it several times for its healing qualities and to bring you in touch with a sense of the sacred embodied in the sex center.

Sit opposite each other in a comfortable position, with your naked genitals easily accessible. You will be holding your own genitals in turn and allowing them to speak through you, in the first person. Each partner will take three turns, for about 5 minutes each time.

This is the type of thing you might say:

Partner 1 "I am the first layer of (name)'s Yoni ... I am like a delicious and delectable fruit who is ever ripe ..." (and so on)

Partner 2 "I am the first layer of (name)'s Lingam ... I am like an antenna, picking up the waves from the Yonis of ovulating women ..." (and so on)

Partner 1 "I am the second layer of (name)'s Yoni. I have secret longings that I would now like to share ..."(and so on)

Partner 2 "I am the second layer of (name)'s Lingam. I am actually very vulnerable, because I need to know that I am loved and respected to be able to function ..." (and so on)

Partner 1 "I am the third layer of (name)'s Yoni. I am the goddess of infinite space. I have no limits ..." (and so on)

Partner 2 "I am the third layer of (name)'s Lingam. I am where God hides. I am actually he who creates life on earth ..." (and so on)

The above gives you an idea of the kind of things that may emerge as you get into the exercise. You don't need to use exactly those words. Just allow your own genitals to speak in a stream-of-consciousness style, without editing or censoring what you say.

♡ Really become your genitals in your imagination. You are not speaking about your genitals – your genitals are speaking through you. You may be very surprised about just how much they have to say.

♡ Do not time each turn exactly – be spontaneous. Around five minutes is usually enough time for each layer to speak.

♡ The three layers of exploration represent the conscious, the subconscious, and the original nature.

♡ You may find that what you express is very different each time you do the exercise. Just trust and allow this process to unfold. Sometimes memories or trauma may come through, in order to be released. If emotion comes up with any layer, just allow the tears and pain to be felt and expressed, to cleanse and renew that layer.

"It was surprising to find that my Yoni had a voice. Layers of feelings came out in different ways – hurt, anger, playfulness, sexiness, longing and beneath them all something wordless: a deep, deep, silent space almost impossible to describe, vast, timeless, sacred, the true essence of my Yoni. As we progressed through the series of these meditations the old layers dropped away and I felt my Yoni become softer, more open, receptive, yielding. Our lovemaking became more beautiful than ever, more expansive, more sacred."

Kamla, Tantra group participant

"It felt somehow risky letting words come out of nowhere: would they be real, or just my imagination? It was like walking off the edge of a cliff and trusting that an invisible hand would place a stepping stone under my feet. And whose invisible hand was offering these stepping stones, these words coming out of the void? I began to feel Kamla's Yoni as a sacred presence communicating with me by a mysterious means. And I more and more began to feel my own Lingam not so much as expressing my sexual energy, but as a gateway for a sacred sexual energy to flow through me."

Andrew, Tantra group participant

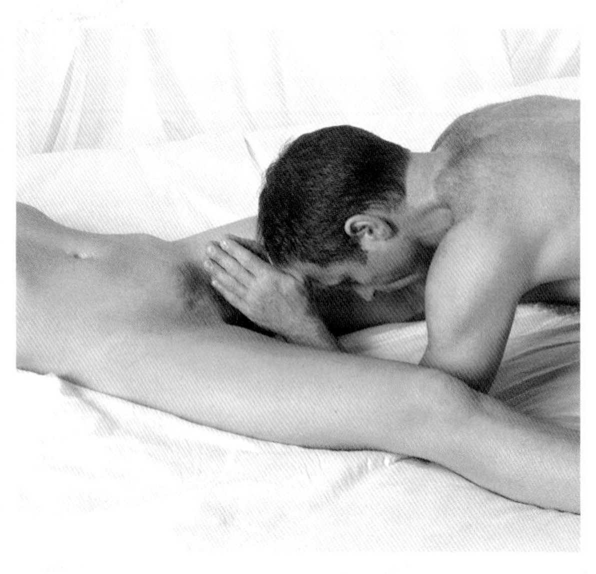

honoring the Yoni

♡ Begin with the man gazing in adoration at the miracle of his beloved's Yoni. Bow down to the goddess principle embodied in this sacred place.

♡ Now become like a bee, drinking nectar from the flower. Use your lips and tongue to pleasure the woman's Yoni, paying special attention to the clitoris. The woman can demonstrate how she likes to be kissed on the Yoni by licking the palm of her partner's hand.

♡ While receiving the honoring of her Yoni, the woman should allow herself to be completely adored as the goddess of love.

♡ The man may enter into a timeless space. If the woman senses that the man is there just for her and has all the time in the world to adore her, she will relax easily into the sublime pleasure that builds up in her whole body as a result of his attention.

Your own sacred place

Focusing on the Yoni and Lingam, suddenly life seems full of promise, for if our bodies contain all the secrets of creation, then certainly godliness is no further away than our own noses. We come very close to godliness when we are in deep rapport with our own genitals, our own sacred place.

Although the genitals are worthy of reverence, many religious teachings have strongly condemned sexual pleasure. Tertullian, one of the founders of orthodox Christianity, said: "Women are the gate by which the demon enters." Perhaps religious teachers feel that if people are in touch with divinity through their bodies, there will be no need for established religions or priests. But if you cut a person off from his or her source of joy, ecstasy, and divine communion they will become lost and confused. You can then step in and become the mediator between them and a distant god high in the heavens, out of reach of mere mortals.

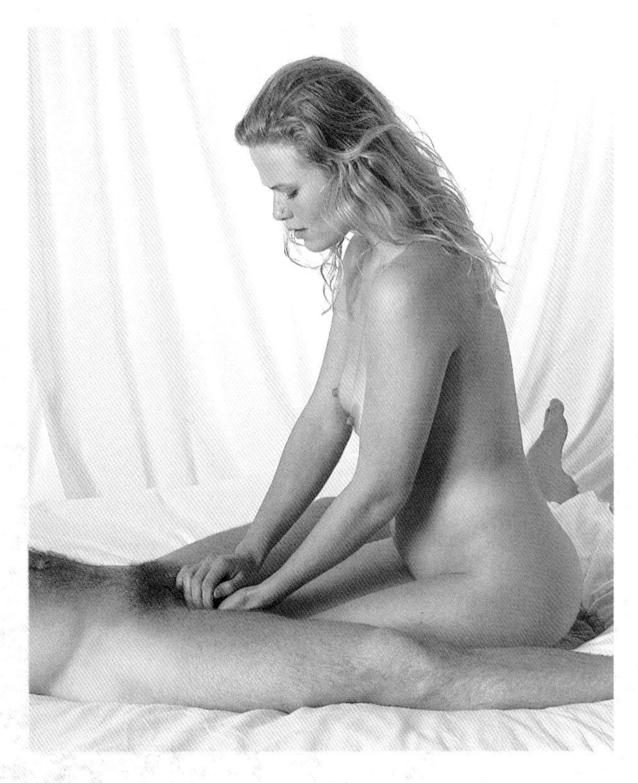

"I felt completely surrendered to the godliness within Ajay and his Lingam, completely losing myself in its power and masculinity.

I felt somehow more empowered, somehow more of a goddess being given the opportunity to express my love in such an intimate way to the man I love. I was at the same time goddess and innocent, seductress and yet humbled."

Mita, Tantra group participant

honoring the Lingam

♡ Begin with the woman holding her partner's soft Lingam in her cupped hands, feeling reverence for the masculine principle.

♡ Gently caress the Lingam and the testicles, and then tenderly take the Lingam in your mouth, just being present with your love. You may like to lick all along the shaft, encouraging arousal, or just to relax, exploring how far you can take the Lingam into your mouth.

♡ Awaken sensation at the perineum, either by licking, by light pressure, or light massage. In Tantra this area is prized as a gateway into higher consciousness. This stimulation will enhance the sensorial experience through the whole body, particularly in the crown chakra (see chapter 8).

♡ The tip of the Lingam has a similar sensitivity to the clitoris. Ask your partner what type of stimulation feels good there. The man can demonstrate by licking and sucking his partner's fingers.

♡ If the erect Lingam becomes like a leaping stallion, it may mean the man is coming close to ejaculation. Some women do not like to receive the ejaculated semen in the mouth; other women adore it. Remember that ejaculation is precious life essence, and treat this moment as sacred.

♡ Taoist Tantra texts recommend that the woman receives the man's ejaculation on her face and breasts and massages it into her skin as a rejuvenating substance. She is then advised to enter into deep meditation as her body absorbs the precious fluid.

The Lingam

"Behold the Shiva Lingam, beautiful as molten gold, firm as the Himalayan Mountain, tender as a folded leaf, life-giving like the solar orb, behold the charm of his sparkling jewels!"
Linga Purana, translated by Nik Douglas

"The universe is the issue of the relationship between a masculine and a feminine principle. Everything, as a result, carries the signature of the Lingam and the Yoni. It is the deity, who in the form of the individual phallus, penetrates each womb and procreates all beings."

From *Karpatri*, translated by Alain Danielou

Lingam means literally "pillar of light" and is the Sanskrit word for the phallus and the exalted male principle. It offers dignity and respect to the penis, and is far removed from words used in common speech. The Lingam is pure life-force energy, the supreme potential creative power. The symbol of the Lingam is worshipped throughout India in temples and in nature, as the manifesting power of Shiva. In the temple, the rounded conical stone representing the phallus rests in a sculpted Yoni. It stands in the centre of the room, proudly proclaiming from its position to be the axis not only of the temple, but also of the world.

Lingam can also mean "sign" or "symbol". When the Lingam moves from its passive soft state to its erect state, it is a sign that the creative force is ready to ignite life. When erect, it throbs with divine energy, awesome to behold. But the Lingam is not only a creative force in producing life on earth; it is also a powerful device for awakening consciousness, elevating men and women to a state of godliness.

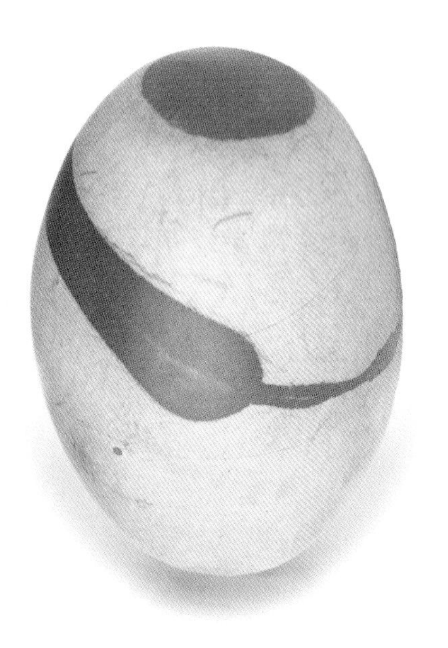

The energy around the sexual organs and in the pelvic region builds up slowly through bodily functions and sits in the pelvis, where it supplies the life force to the reproductive organs and glands. In Yoga or Tantra this energy is called Kundalini, and is represented in its dormant state as a coiled snake. Sex is the most potent way of awakening Kundalini energy, which "uncoils" from its dormant state and is released through ejaculation (in the male) or rises in the spine (in either male or female) opening new levels of ecstasy, bliss, and consciousness.

The symbol of the Lingam as a pillar of light can be found throughout the world, from Asia and Africa to Europe, the Americas and Australia. Ancient symbols include standing stones, sculpted rounded stones, or pointed conical pillars. Today the symbol of the phallus can be seen in the obelisks in many towns and cities in the world. As it is an axis of power, if the phallus is positioned alone, without the balancing influence of a Yoni to rest in, it can be used to unleash negative controlling energies. In balanced societies Lingam worship is balanced by Yoni worship, to ensure harmony in society.

The anatomy of the Lingam

The Lingam serves a dual function. In its passive resting state, urine is released through a hole at its tip. When the Lingam is in its aroused, erect state, semen is expelled through the same hole. Both cannot happen at the same time. We can only marvel at the intricacy of its design.

"In the midst of the subtle center situated at the body's lowest point, said to be a triangle whose three sides are desire, knowledge, action, rises that Lingam born of itself and glowing like a thousand suns."

Shiva Purana, Tantra chronicle

At puberty the testes produce an abundance of testosterone, a hormone that brings with it the male attributes of size, muscle tone, bone mass, strength, and abundant libido. The sexually mature male produces about 300 million sperm per day, which are stored in the seminal duct. If no ejaculation occurs, the body will reabsorb the stored sperm after a period of one month.

When the Lingam becomes erect, the foreskin recedes along the shaft, enhancing the full glory of the Lingam unveiled, like a sudden burst of sun as it rises in the morning. The erection of the Lingam is an area of great interest and bewilderment to both men and women. Its physiological functioning has been clearly explained by science and can even be provoked using drugs, but this does not explain fully the range of experiences of erection a man can have. Every man knows that a single thought can bring an erection, but so can stimulus through the different senses: seeing a naked woman in your bed, watching an erotic scene in a movie, hearing "love sounds" and "love words", or smelling a particular scent. Rubbing or touching the Lingam is a common way to bring arousal, but still the Lingam seems to have a mind of its own.

The Lingam also responds to the bio-electrical pull of a woman's Yoni that is fully ready. This is a different arousal mechanism from thoughts or stimulation through the senses. When the body is relaxed, erection will come without any effort the moment the Yoni is ready to invite the Lingam in. It is an art in Tantra to wait for the right moment and prepare a woman for penetration and it is then that the Lingam can become easily and naturally erect.

Tantra sees the prostate gland as a relay station for conveying the soul to sexual expression. The life force, or Kundalini energy is accessed at the prostate, allowing the man to draw from a never-ending source of energy. This increases his sexual potency and gives him the possibility of experiencing powerful spiritual states of consciousness. Accessing and preserving this energy is the reason behind the Tantric practice of retention of ejaculation, or re-absorption of vital energy. The prostate gland is the "soul" of the man's sexuality. Therefore it will be affected negatively if the man suffers from too much or not enough ejaculation, or psychological imbalances around his sexuality.

Circumcision

Circumcision is the practice of cutting off the foreskin. In some cultures baby boys are circumcised either for religious or hygiene reasons. Many men in the world remain uncircumcised with no ill effect, so hygiene is not the key issue, but young boys need to be taught how to wash the Lingam. Over time, as the foreskin becomes free, it should be gently pulled back for daily washing, which can become a very pleasurable experience!

Some people think that because circumcised men have less sensitivity in the crown of the Lingam, they are able to make love for a longer time. In fact, the more sensitivity he has, the more the man can feel the delicate bio-electric currents that pass between Yoni and Lingam, so he can be a more responsive lover. Each boy should be given the right to decide for himself whether or not he would like such an operation performed, when he comes of age. However, if you are already circumcised, do not worry. You can develop an all-over body sensitivity, which will bring profound fulfilment (see page 46).

Union of Lingam and Yoni

Lingam and Yoni in union promote health and wellbeing. The genitals contain acupressure points related to the organs, so each loving act of sex between male and female partners is also an acupressure healing session for the whole body/mind.

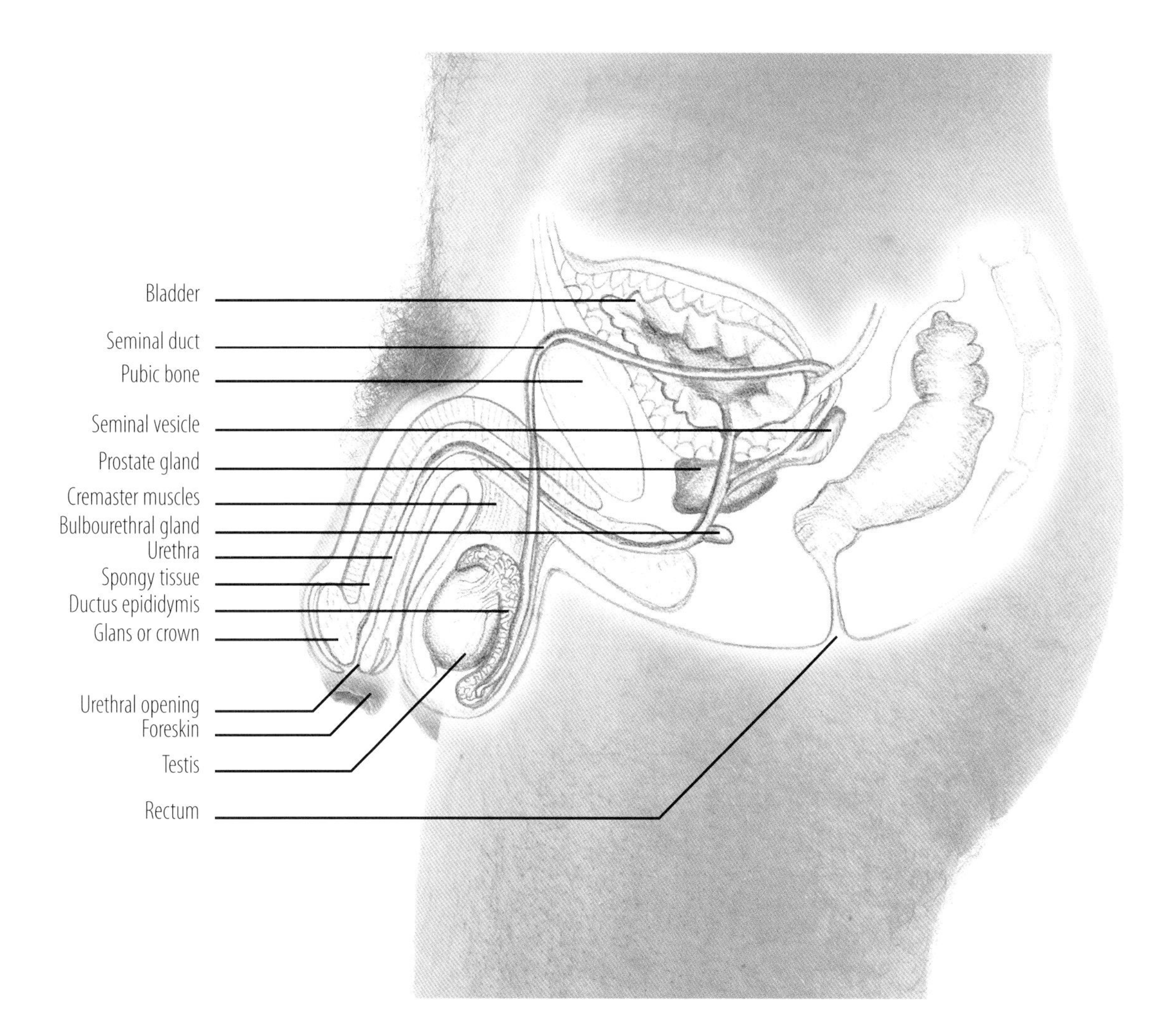

Arteries and spongy tissue inside the shaft become engorged with blood to create an erection.

Urethra: tube through which urine and semen flow.

Glans or crown: the tip of the Lingam.

Foreskin: covers and protects the crown when the Lingam is in its resting state.

Testicles: hang outside the body to keep sperm at optimum temperature. In the cold, they are pulled closer to the body for warmth, by the Cremaster muscles.

Ductus epididymis: 20 feet of tubes coiled inside the testicles, where sperm mature for 10–14 days before moving to the seminal duct.

Seminal duct: where sperm are stored.

Prostate gland: releases prostatic fluid, which gives semen its milky appearance and brings mobility and nutrients to the sperm.

Seminal vesicle: releases seminal fluid, which mixes with prostatic fluid and sperm to form semen.

chapter 3

head and pelvis communication

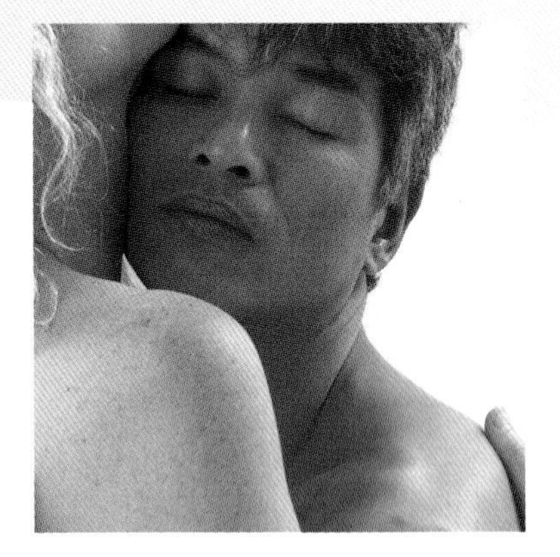

"I hold your head right
Between my thighs and press
Against your mouth and
Float away forever in
An orchid boat
On the river of Heaven."
Marichiko (Japanese Love Poem)

The communication network in the human body is a fascinating subject. For a deeper understanding of it, we need to look into the beginning: the embryo in the womb. The embryo's genetic blueprint determines how it develops physically, and in the same way its energetic blueprint governs its emotional development. It is the programming that the foetus receives from its environment that establishes this energetic blueprint.

"Place your whole attention in the nerve,
delicate as the lotus thread,
in the centre of your spinal column,
in such be transformed."

Vigyan Bhairav Tantra, Shiva

Experiences before birth

At the beginning of the embryo's life, the moment of conception programs the experience of sex into the energetic blueprint. If the moment of conception is ecstatic, the embryo receives a celebrative imprint of sexuality. Once the mother knows that she is pregnant, how she receives the news will also affect the embryo. If the mother is welcoming to the new being, then the child will be able to move forward in life in a relaxed way, knowing that he or she is welcomed by existence. If the mother is horrified, in denial, or considering abortion, the child will carry with him or her a feeling of being a burden, unwanted by life.

After three to four weeks in the womb, the embryo's spine and vertebral canal has formed, the heart has started beating, and other body systems are developing. From now, all the different imprints the embryo receives are recorded in the spine, which then feeds the information into the organs. At eight weeks' gestation the brain is developed, so from then on the mother's intellectual stimulus will also affect the foetus. In particular the foetus will recognize music that it hears regularly. It has been found that if a mother regularly watches a soap opera on TV, her baby will recognize the theme tune of that soap opera after birth, and may find it calming and reassuring. At 14 weeks, the heart center opens. If the child is welcomed and loved he or she will receive an imprint that life is love, which will help all his or her future relationships.

At 20 weeks, the center of power in the solar plexus opens. For the first six months of the pregnancy, the developing child is not fully committed to staying in the womb. In a sense it is "testing the water" to see if this is the correct choice of womb. When the center of power opens, this helps to anchor the child to its personal choice in bonding with this mother and the life that awaits. From now on, the child will more easily adapt to the ups and downs which life brings. Before the center of power opens, if something shocking happens the foetus can more easily miscarry. Shocks may include physical or psychological violence, negative emotional states, accidents to the mother, smoking, or ingestion of chemicals in drugs or processed foods.

By around 26 to 27 weeks in the womb, the mother's attitude toward giving birth strongly affects the child. If the mother is terrified of labour and birth, her terror communicates to the child that taking a step into the unknown is dangerous. In adult life, the child may become a person who fears each change that life brings. If the mother is relaxed and joyous, able to welcome the transition into birth, this will give the baby a positive outlook, that life's challenges are to be welcomed. An experienced midwife and antenatal classes, ideally for both parents, can do wonders in alleviating pre-birth fears.

At the birth, if the mother is drugged this will give the imprint that drugs are needed to cope with life. If the mother is able to move consciously and celebratively with the birth process, this will inspire a deep "yes" for life in the child.

The energy pathway

The spine is a very delicate networking system that links the brain with the pelvis; it is an energy pathway between sex and spirit. As we have seen, experiences before birth are imprinted in the spine. Throughout life, trauma or shock will also affect the spine, and be revealed as pain, abnormal curvatures, or tensions.

This is one reason why massage and other types of bodywork are so valuable. They can help release trauma and inspire a vibrant flow of life energy between head and pelvis. When this energy is flowing, the pleasure a person feels in sex can spread through the whole body. When energy flows freely between head and pelvis, sensitivity is heightened and this leads to ecstatic, spiritually awakened states of being.

"Every individual has encased in his or her skull both a feminine brain and a masculine one. Any particular society can accentuate one or the other of these two ways of interacting with the world, depending on the demands of the environment or the shaping influences of its inventions."

Leonard Shlain
The Alphabet vs the Goddess

Because the brain and the sexual organs are linked closely through the spine's communication network, many holistic therapies such as acupuncture, color light therapy, and shiatsu use points on the genitals to treat ailments of the head, and vice versa. The theory behind craniosacral therapy is that the brain and spinal cord more or less control the entire nervous system, and the pituitary and pineal glands and hypothalamus govern the endocrine system and the hormones it secretes, so treating the head and spinal areas will have a powerful effect over a wide variety of bodily functions. Many women have discovered that one of the best cures for migraine is a few orgasms.

Systems in the brain

The glandular and nervous systems of the brain are like little kingdoms in the empire of the body/mind and are of paramount importance in the overall functioning of our sexuality and well-being. The hypothalamus governs the production of hormones and the will to live and procreate, and is the primary element in any mind-over-body type of experience. It works in concert with the pituitary gland, which rules over sexual desire, the endocrine system, and some emotional states. The pineal gland, known as the gland of light, rules over sleeping and waking patterns and also influences the awakening of intuition and clairvoyance.

The thalamus is a principal relay station for sensory impulses travelling along the spinal cord and into the brain. It also interprets these impulses, checking them against memory records from previous experiences. If you have suffered trauma from a sensory experience, your thalamus will need loving attention in order to release this and be open to the new. The thalamus is also a gateway into higher states of consciousness.

The corpus callosum is very important to your sexual being, because it is the link between the right and left hemispheres of the brain. The right hemisphere of the brain controls the left hand side of the body and rules over the dimensions of creativity, imagination, dream states, intuition, and music. It is more female in its orientation, and in tune with being. Conversely, the left hemisphere of the brain controls the right hand side of the body and rules over logic, mathematics, analysis, speaking, and the principle of doing. It is more male in aspect. In Tantra, the ultimate attainment is the conscious and balanced merging of the inner male and female aspects through the corpus callosum.

The most exalted qualities of these brain systems can be discovered through the practice of sacred sexuality. Sacred sexuality involves learning to meditate, or bring awareness to the sex act and male–female dynamics. It means creating a sacred space in which sex takes on a divine quality.

The flow of sexual energy

When sexual energy is not allowed to flow freely, it creates confusion in the natural energy flow. The sexual energy has nowhere to express itself but through the mind, and this can lead eventually to obsessive mental sexuality and perversion. Twisted sexual energy arising from repression can also lead to mental, emotional, and physical disease. When we allow the natural energy flow between head and pelvis, there is a discharge of neuropeptides – pleasure hormones – which activate joy in being alive, and thus support health and longevity.

In the ancient Eastern cultures of India, China, Tibet, and Japan, the practice of sexuality was honed to a fine art and utilized for physical health and spiritual awakening. In these traditions the link between head and pelvis is Kundalini energy. Kundalini Yoga and Tantra both teach a science of evolution whereby the practitioner can utilize raw sexual energy, raising it up through the spinal column, leading to an orgasmic state of awakened consciousness. If sexual energy is repressed, then a person has no fuel for such an experience. Only when sexuality is accepted and explored in freedom and with sensitivity and intelligence can it then be channelled into higher consciousness.

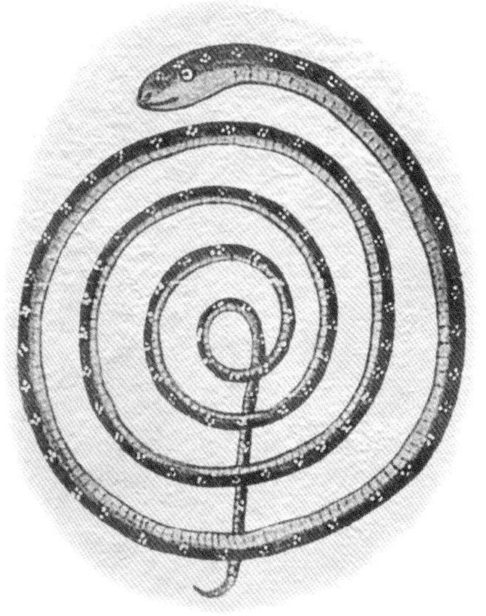

The power of raw sexual energy and our spiritual potential is represented by the symbol of the serpent coiled at the base of the spine.

opening the sex and spirit connection

♡ A simple way of opening the sex and spirit connection is to exchange a massage with your lover, touching points on the sacrum that are directly linked to the glandular system of the brain (see diagram, opposite).

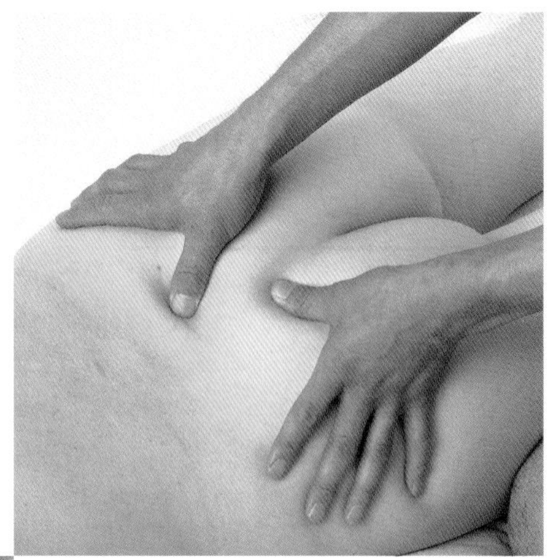

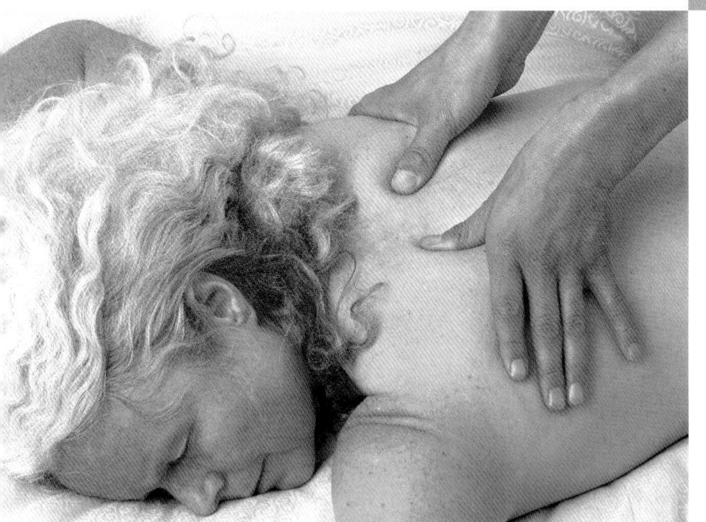

♡ Then use your hands to move the energy that has been awakened in the sacrum up along either side of the spine. This allows the neuropeptides, called encephalins, to release their pleasure-giving qualities. When you reach the top of the spine, move this energy through the shoulders and out through the arms and hands.

♡ Massaging around the area in the centre of the back between the underarm folds will also free the energy flow in the genitals.

♡ Complete this massage by simultaneously touching the perineum, the point between the sex organs and anus (an important acupuncture point known as Hui Yin) and the top of the head, or crown chakra (see page 78). This affirms the link between the head and the pelvis – heaven and earth inside the body.

♡ While in the sex act, to deepen intimacy and to bring an expansion of consciousness to your union, allow your foreheads to connect at the level of the eyebrows. This stimulates the pineal gland, helping to awaken the third eye (see page 78). This will give a much more free-flowing, ecstatic quality to your lovemaking.

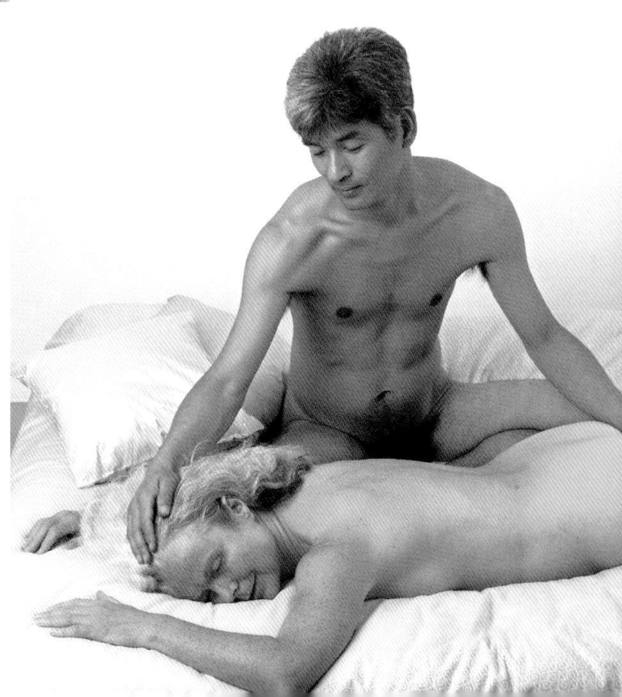

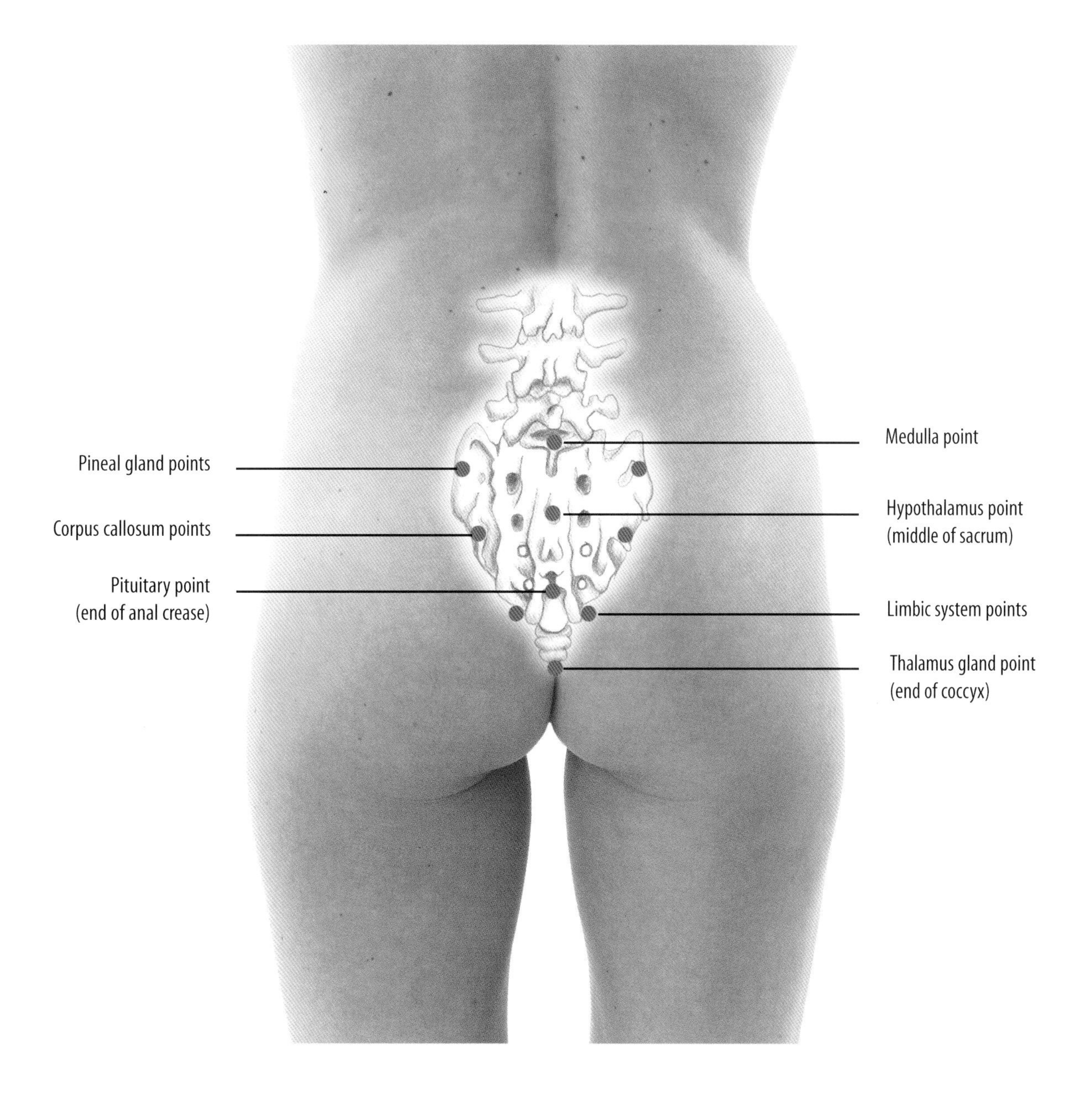
Medulla point
Pineal gland points
Hypothalamus point
(middle of sacrum)
Corpus callosum points
Pituitary point
(end of anal crease)
Limbic system points
Thalamus gland point
(end of coccyx)

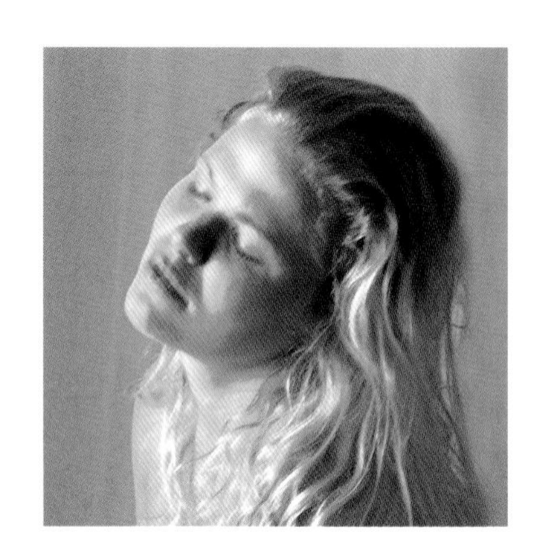

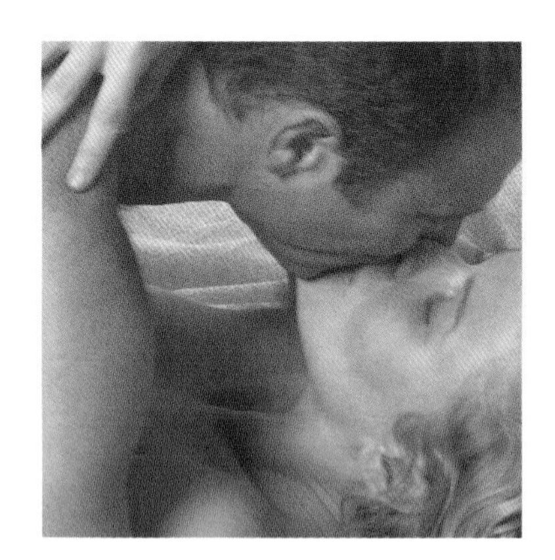

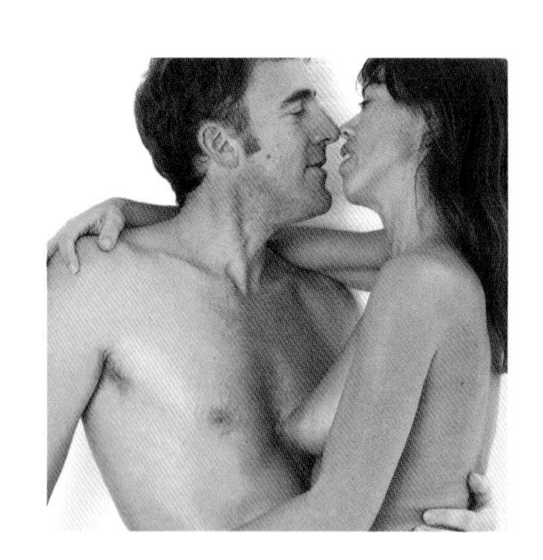

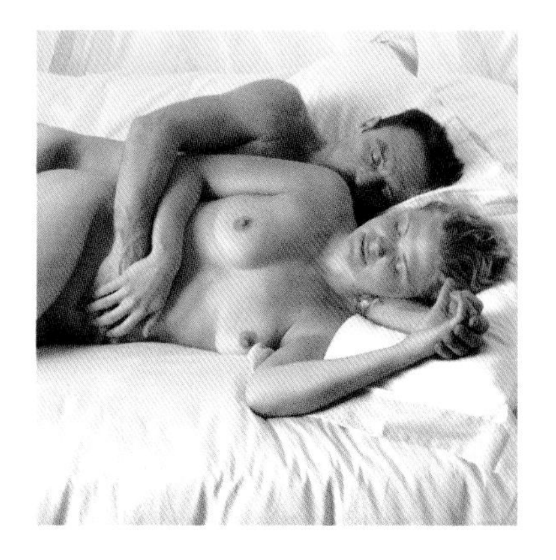

part 2
sex

Sex is the origin of all the beauties of our world. Through the sexual interaction of all living things, we see godliness at work. Therefore the sex act deserves our highest regard and most profound research.

Pleasure is the key to the tremendous teaching inherent in sex, and understanding orgasm intimately is a prerequisite for a fulfilled life. Self-pleasuring is a natural and enjoyable way to understand our own capacity for orgasmic states of being. It gives empowering self-knowledge for sexual union with a partner. With a deep acceptance of sex and orgasm as a diving board into a celebrative, spiritual lifestyle, merging with a lover is a deeply rewarding experience.

Imagine living an orgasmic life in an orgasmic world. This is not such a far-off possibility. It is all about remembering and accessing the key contained in orgasm and using this key to open the door of life. You will find it fits perfectly – they were made for each other. As we allow a sensual sensitivity to flow all over the body, we can enhance the practical knowledge of how sex functions with our own deep experience, making us wise, joyous, and free.

chapter 4

self-pleasuring

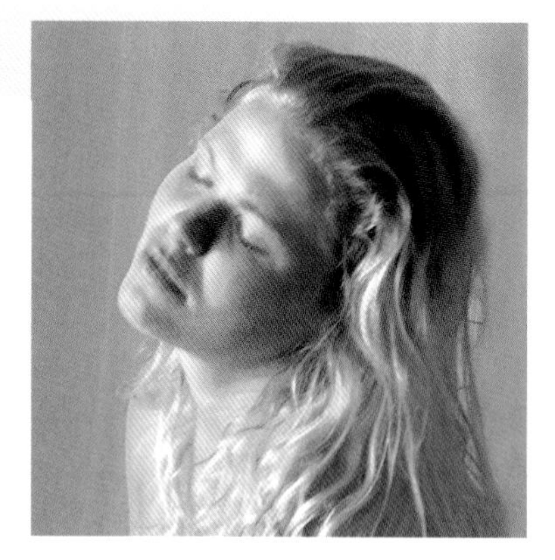

"Self pleasuring, for both men and women, is a kind of apprenticeship. It's an important source of self awareness – a prerequisite to being good in bed."
From *Manhood*, by Steve Biddulph

Female self-pleasuring

The intimate discovery of your body is truly the royal road to a fulfilled life. Unimpeded sexual revelation happens in the private moments of what is usually called masturbation. The term self-pleasuring is softer on the tongue.

In an ideal world, as a girl grows up she will be allowed freedom to explore her body, without shame or censure. In this way she will naturally discover for herself, in her own time, the body movements and types of self-pleasuring touch that fill her with delight.

"Letting go into myself,
Riding waves
Getting bigger and bigger
Experiencing a stillness
And then more waves.
The more I let go, the bigger I become."

Female Tantra group participant

When Shere Hite was researching into female sexuality for *The Hite Report* (1976) and *The New Hite Report* (2000), she found that the self-pleasuring techniques a girl uses when she is young establish how she will respond sexually as an adult. For example, some women have discovered self-pleasure as young girls by moving rhythmically up and down on a bunched-up blanket. As adults, they employ the same type of movement to come to orgasm on top of a man. Another type of woman has learned self-pleasuring by lying down on her back, legs spread, caressing her clitoris. She will continue to need this type of stimulation in order to orgasm while making love with a man. Yet another type of woman has learned pleasuring by squeezing her thighs together very hard and stimulating her clitoris by internal squeezing of the genital muscles. She will continue to require this type of stimulation with a lover.

In other words, how you respond sexually as an adult depends a lot on how you have trained yourself to respond to pleasurable sensations as a child. If your childhood was one where you were not given the space physically or psychologically in which to explore your body, you will need to give yourself that space to reclaim your right to pleasure.

In this context, it is important not to judge yourself. Some women think their genitals are ugly or smell bad, or they think the desire for orgasm is wrong, or that they should reach orgasm in a different way than they do. All these kinds of judgements are really conditioning that you have absorbed from others. You were not born with such ideas. Newborn babies and young children have no shame, inhibitions, or self-judgements. Let yourself be reborn in your exploration of self-pleasuring.

Some women may like to use mechanical pleasuring devices such as a vibrator and or dildo to attain orgasm. This is a good way to initiate confidence that orgasm is possible for you. However, it is wise not to over-use such devices, or you will be training your body to require that amount of mechanical stimulation in order to orgasm. It may then become more and more difficult to come to orgasm easily and naturally with a lover. No man can compete with a machine, and if you are addicted to the machine then you may miss many of the subtle nuances of pleasure that arise with a human lover. Also, a dildo made of a hard unyielding substance may damage the delicate Yoni. If you wish to use a dildo it is preferable to use something natural and pliable such as a peeled cucumber (cucumber cleanses and rejuvenates the Yoni). After initiating orgasm with a vibrator, come back to human touch and find out how to reach even higher peaks with movement and touch alone.

"When I was 12 years old, my elder sister suggested that I take a bath and spread my legs under the warm running tap water. When I asked her why, she merely smiled and said, "You'll find out!" So I tried it and experienced my first orgasm. After that I became quite addicted to baths!

When I started having sex with men I could not have orgasm with them. In order to be satisfied I had to have a bath! It was not until I was 17 and living in India, where bathtubs were rare, that I began training myself to become more sensitive to other ways of coming to orgasm.

To do this I had to return to a state of innocence and discover my body again, as if for the first time. As part of this process I even went so far as to enjoy a honeymoon with myself, self-pleasuring non-stop for three days! This gave me a heightened sensitivity where orgasm with men became possible."

Sarita

Becoming an empress of love

When you know the art of pleasuring yourself, you will become empowered in the sex act with a man. If you enter the sex act not knowing what brings you to orgasm, but hoping the man will do some magic to take you there, you are placing yourself in a weak position that will usually lead to frustration with the lover. Knowing your own body, knowing the time you need, the style you like, and what ecstasy you are capable of, will make you an empress of love. Old Victorian ideas have taught generations of women that it is wrong to seek our own pleasure, that a "lady" simply accommodates the man for his pleasure. Let us throw out these outdated ideas and celebrate the return of the empress of love. A real "lady" is a woman who is fully orgasmic.

celebrate being a woman

♡ Make an appointment with yourself, for about one hour, twice a week. This is your sacred time of self-discovery. Make sure you will not be disturbed during this time.

♡ During your self-discovery time, begin by pretending that you are a young girl again. Imagine your age as you begin softly to caress your naked body, finding out about it in total innocence. Who am I in a young girl's body? Where are my pleasure zones? What brings me delight? At this stage, there is no need to reach a sexual climax. It is simply a time of exploration.

♡ As you continue with your appointments, go on growing up slowly in your imagination.

♡ When you come to the age of puberty your exploration may become more overtly sexual. Take a mirror and look closely into your genital area. Pull back the hood of your clitoris and examine it. Open your vaginal lips and look at the beautiful folds and colors. See the opening of your vagina, the sacred channel for new life to be born. Explore inside with your fingers, smell and taste your essence.

♡ Write a poem about your experience.

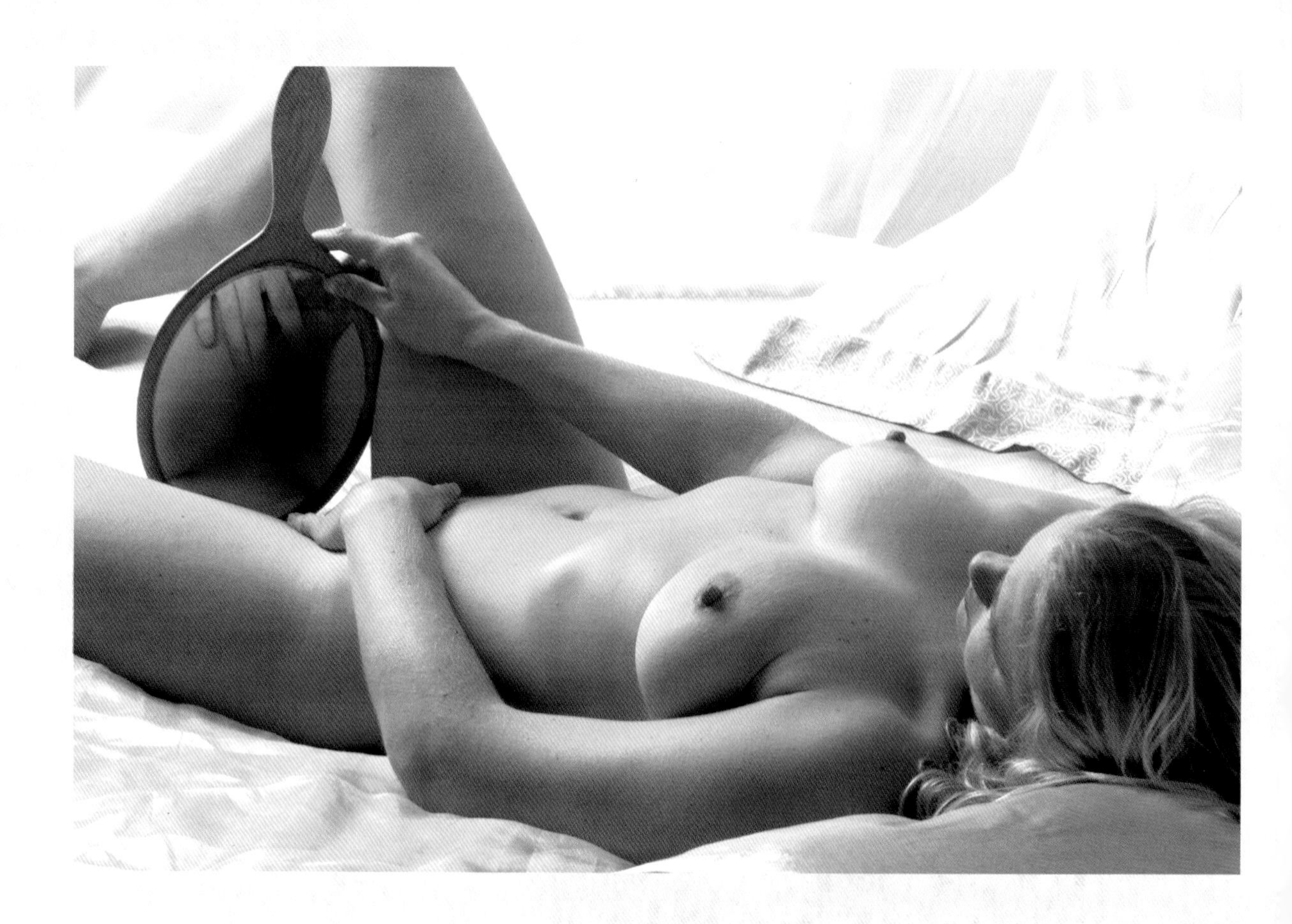

♡ Continue your sensual journey. There is no need to be in a hurry. Just continue your regular appointments and keep adding new areas of discovery. Find out how many pleasure spots you have in your body. Caress your breasts, your face, your lips, your ears, your anus. (Be aware, if you insert a finger into your anus, do not then insert the same finger into your vagina, or you may spread bacteria that can lead to a urinary tract infection.) Know your whole body as a garden of delight.

♡ Start experimenting with different body positions. Which bring more sensual pleasure? Touch your genitals in different ways, rubbing, squeezing, stroking and caressing in different rhythms.

♡ Let fantasy take hold of you. Imagine yourself with a lover and how you wish to know your body through physical contact.

♡ Discover intimately how you best experience the build-up toward orgasm. Do you need steady and rhythmic stimulation to your clitoris or mount of Venus? Or do you enjoy a varied pattern, a teasing slow build-up to the crescendo? Do you feel more pleasure with your fingers inside your vagina? Do you enjoy one or more orgasms? Do you need your breasts touched for a full-body build-up?

♡ Find out which times of the moon cycle invite you into states of heightened pleasure.

♡ To help free and open your mind so that you can experience maximum pleasure without inhibition, allow yourself to make all kinds of sounds and body movements. Try roaring like a lioness, laughing like a hyena, or operatic singing during your orgasmic states. Be completely abandoned into the river of love. Celebrate being a woman. Consider yourself a goddess.

enhancing love play with self-pleasuring

It is a very enriching experience to practice self-pleasuring while with a lover.

♡ Take the time to lie down one at a time, in front of each other, and enter into self-pleasuring. Let your lover see all the nuances of touch and the qualities of build-up you enjoy.

♡ It is better not to talk during your sexual play, so as not to leak the energy from what you are experiencing.

♡ When you have moved into orgasm, hold each other and share that beautiful and intimate space together.

♡ When you are ready, you can exchange roles.

♡ Afterward, share what you have learned from each other. This will bring a great depth of understanding to your love union.

Male self-pleasuring

Self-pleasuring starts very early in life. It is now known that the foetus in the mother's womb touches its genitals. After birth a boy goes on feeling the need to touch his genitals. He does so because it is comforting and is also a valuable way for him to discover the life force in his body.

"My genitals light up
Brighter and brighter and brighter
Then suddenly a dazzling fulfilment
Exploding into the whole body
That rises up and takes over"

Male Tantra group participant

When a baby boy is put into nappies, he is prevented from accessing his genitals and his anus. In this way from the very outset of his life he is deprived of something that makes him feel relaxed and filled with pleasure.

A friend told us how when her child was small, she had all the floors in her apartment covered with linoleum and let the child run around with a bare bottom, cleaning up when necessary. In many areas of India, babies do not wear nappies – the mother simply knows the right moment to take the child outside. This is not to say that nappies are wrong, but a balance is good. Whenever possible, give a child a little time to play naked and free of any restrictions.

A baby boy has no negative conditioning around his genitals. Touching his genitals activates his root chakra, thus helping the inner circular flow of energy, which will connect his sex center through the vertical channel inside the body with the crown chakra at the top of his head (see page 78). In that vertical flow, he is whole, at one with himself and with all that is; a deep sense of wellbeing surrounds him. This is a mystical state of being. The circulation of energy will also promote brain function and lymph flow. Because of the ecstasy he experiences, the boy will take deep breaths, leading to greater oxygenation of the blood and more vibrant life in his body.

A child is naturally in the state of being which we could call paradise on earth. The remembrance of this state of being remains in the adult's psyche as a deep unspoken longing that carries an almost religious significance. Mystics down the ages have talked about returning to the innocence of the child or having a second birth.

The mother or father cleaning the boy's bottom and genitals should do so with tender loving care and appreciation, as this will create a positive imprint that the boy will carry toward this part of his body. If the parent finds cleaning the child disgusting or distasteful, this message will taint the boy's relationship with his own genitals, and he will carry it over as an imprint into his adulthood. As he grows up, the boy may often receive the message that it is not socially correct to touch his genitals. This idea will contribute to his gradual disconnection with that flow of energy in his body.

Around puberty, hormonal changes propel the boy into a new discovery: ejaculation. Ejaculation is exciting, the culmination of a very intense build-up of energy in the genitals, and a completely new experience. For the boy it is not sexual, it is just a new discovery, a new possibility the body is suddenly offering, just like that, out of the blue.

This new pleasure reconnects him with his genitals. He will mainly use this hormonal momentum to provoke genital release through ejaculation. If in the past he has received negative messages about touching his genitals, he no longer knows the art of touching his genitals to simply come home and reconnect his energy to the whole. He does it hurriedly and furtively, so that nobody finds out his new secret. This hurried way of self-pleasuring becomes habitual and does not leave much room for loving, sensual awakening of his energy. This habit creates a pattern that will be carried into his sex life with women. Many men stay in that pattern their whole lives, never becoming aware of the great heights and depths that sex can offer.

Love is the bridge

Touching our own genitals is a very natural and healthy practice. We have to re-learn how to do so sensitively, to provoke a circulation of energy that will re-open the possibilities we once knew as a baby. The way to reconnect with that experience is through love. Through love a man can access a deep feeling of wellbeing. The common experience of male self-pleasuring is a poor substitute for the ecstatic experience that Tantra describes as orgasm. It is every man's birthright to know this type of expansive, whole-body orgasmic experience. Love is the bridge: through love the man moves from sex into an emotional and spiritual connection to his own body and the whole of existence.

love yourself as a man

While touching his genitals, a man can enter into a space of loving himself, with so much love that his body energies start to open and circulate freely.

The "normal" way of self-pleasuring to ejaculation does not open a flow of energy around the sex center. It is a more or less mechanical method of bringing about ejaculation in a predictable sequence. There is nothing wrong with this type of sexual experience, if that is what is desired at that moment. However, if that is the only way the man knows of experiencing his sexuality, he will be missing the expansive pleasure that is possible when he allows his sexual energy to spread all over his body.

♡ Touch the Lingam and testicles and around the genitals (including between the testicles and the anus) with great love and joy, to awaken the energies around the pelvis.

♡ As you continue to focus on loving and enjoying yourself, then the build-up of energy will flood your lower belly. You may need to let sounds out: moaning, roaring, or other sounds that express your longing for total orgasm. Making these sounds opens your second chakra (see page 78) and you will start to feel delirious.

♡ To allow the energies to burst through the solar plexus, move your body, snaking your spine, arching your back, and flow into other movements and positions that come spontaneously. Whether or not you are touching your genitals at this point is irrelevant. Let go and give your body complete freedom to move in ecstasy.

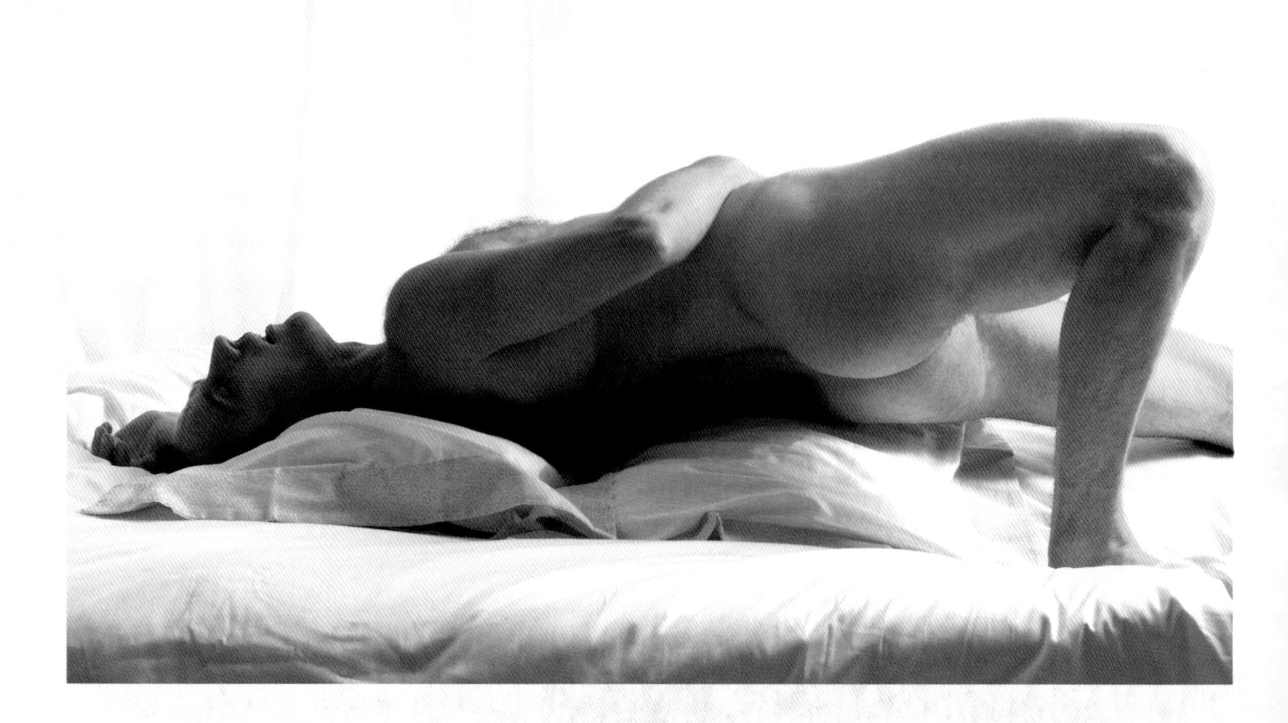

♡ This will lead you to the first reward: orgasm of the heart. You will know at this point that sex and heart are part of the same energy, the union of your own complementary male and female aspects. You will discover what ecstasy is.

♡ This experience can be emotional, perhaps bringing with it anger or tears or laughter. Do not reject those aspects of your energy; allow them to be part of your love session in that moment. Then you can go beyond them to a cosmic experience of sex.

♡ Imagine that you are making love to the universe, penetrating the cosmic Yoni and being wholly swallowed. That is what we mean by "becoming orgasmic". You lose yourself completely. You become orgasm itself.

♡ By allowing yourself to become orgasmic in this way you may find that whether you ejaculate or not is irrelevant. The intensity of pleasure has found a new pathway. Let this be a sacred time to discover your full potential as a man.

♡ This experience will make you a master lover. You will know the feminine experience from inside yourself and there will be no separation between you and a woman. By loving yourself like this, you will know the greatest secrets of sex. Yang moves into Yin and Yin moves back into Yang in an infinite loop, which has no beginning and no ending.

"At 15 I had a lot of excess sexual energy but felt that ejaculation ended things just when it was getting good. I found that by taking deep slow breaths to relax my whole body and changing the sexual stimulation to a very light shake of the hand, while massaging my chest and nipples with the other, I was able to maintain my pleasure and yet avoid coming. It was like finding a secret path around the inevitable ending, into a spacious and luminous inner world. My penis would jerk and spasm as if releasing tension but with no coming. I could then safely increase the intensity of touch to enjoy waves of wonderful pleasure long into the night."

Male Tantra group participant

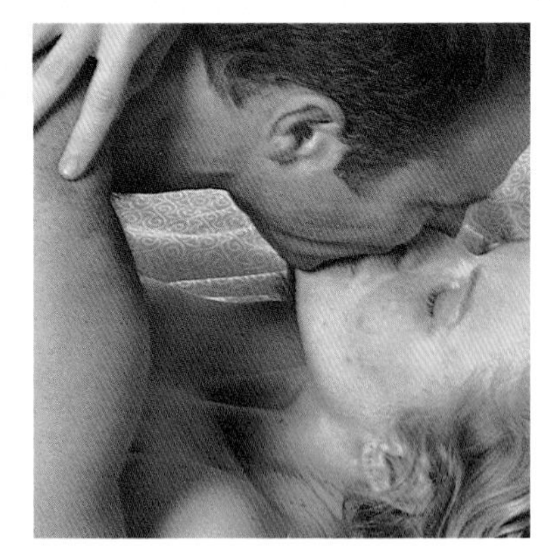

orgasm

"Kiss me again, rekiss me, kiss me more,
give me your most consuming, tasty one
Give me your sensual kiss, a savoury one,
I'll give you four back, burning at the core
Are you up in arms?
Well, I'll give you ten erotic kisses for your appetite
And we will mingle kisses and excite our bodies
with an easy joy again."
French love poem, Louise Labe (1524–66)

"I scream, and laugh, and cry.
The rest of the world disappears.
I explode, I am no more.
Everything becomes vast.
Time and mind disappear.
And within this, an incredible sense of presence
a presence of the divine."

Female Tantra group participant

The nature of orgasm takes us beyond time and mind. It is a moment of absolute disappearance of oneself, being overtaken by something bigger, vaster than ourselves. It is a letting go into the mysteries of existence, and so highly spiritual. Tantra recognizes the spirituality of orgasm and understands that it contains the key to human potential, the ultimate orgasm with the universe. Sexual orgasm hints at the possibility of applying orgasmic qualities to everyday life, learning to live as an ecstatic being. It is time for us to relearn that capacity, and thereby transform our lives on this earth into paradise.

Male or Yang energy is an active, outward-going impulse that seeks expression. It is like a straight line that goes directly to the point. Female or Yin energy follows a more curved path. It is interesting to observe that a man's body does not usually have as many curves as a woman's body, and his erect Lingam shows beautifully how the Yang aspect of life seeks direct expression.

Female orgasm

According to research by sex therapists, the build-up for female orgasm is fed from whole-body arousal. During this build-up, or foreplay, which may take 20 minutes or more, both the interior and exterior parts of the female genitals become engorged and enlarged to perhaps twice their usual size. The vagina expands like a balloon, becoming longer and wider, and there may be copious secretions. In some women the ballooning of the vagina creates a strong desire for penetrative sex.

The clitoris is the focal center for pleasure during foreplay, becoming erect as the build-up occurs. The 3000 nerve endings in the clitoris are all devoted to pleasure, and are linked to erogenous zones all over the body. The build-up of pleasure in and around the clitoris may happen through direct physical stimulation of the clitoris itself, or through stimulation of other parts of the body. Some women may experience orgasm simply through having their breasts massaged. This is because nerves located in the nipples have a direct link to the clitoris. Also, these nerve links ensure that the pleasure a woman feels in foreplay will involve the whole of her body/mind.

As the build-up continues, the breasts swell, nipples and clitoris become erect, and the labia minora swell and become flushed. Breathing rate, heart rate, and blood pressure all increase. At the moment of orgasm a spinal reflex in the area of the sacrum sends sympathetic nerve impulses to the circum vaginal and perineal muscles, giving rise to rhythmic contractions at 0.8-second intervals. These contractions engulf the woman in waves of ecstatic release. This is an automatic reflex, not a voluntary one, meaning it does not depend on will to function. However, if she is not relaxed, the woman's will can inhibit the orgasm reflex, suppressing this release. This can lead to a build-up of nervous tension, migraines, and similar problems. Conversely, your conscious participation in the process of orgasm can enhance its effect, if you are open, flowing with your energy and emotions, and able to let go of control.

Although the basic body mechanics for orgasm are always the same, the intensity of orgasm varies from woman to woman, and also depends on the woman's physcial and mental state at that particular moment. This gave rise to Freud's mistaken belief, since proved wrong, that there are different types of orgasm – a vaginal orgasm and a clitoral orgasm. Freud stated that the vaginal orgasm was superior and belonged to sane and balanced women, while the clitoral orgasm was infantile and belonged to neurotic women. Thus any woman who could not orgasm through penetration alone, but needed clitoral stimulation, was neurotic. This misconception has tortured countless women and prevented them from leading ecstatic sex lives.

Abundant research has disproved Freud's theory. Masters and Johnson, in their 20-year study of human sexual response, found that women who seemingly orgasm from penetration alone are actually actively stimulating their clitoris during this process, though not using hands to do so. Most sex therapists now agree that even during penetrative sex, orgasm is triggered by stimulation of the clitoris. As the Lingam moves rhythmically in the Yoni, it pulls on the labia minora, which are connected to the fold of skin around the clitoris, the clitoral hood. The movements of the clitoral hood, and pressure from the man's pubic bone, stimulate the clitoris directly.

"Opening.
Starts with my heart
Expanding, going out
Through that my sex opens, letting go
Waves through my body
And waves going outwards
Flowing, bobbing on the sea
Feeling a sense of something more
Moving towards a stiller space
Earthy, rooted in my body
Energy coming up from the earth."

Female Tantra group participant

Whole-body arousal

A woman's orgasm will be much more intense if she has time to allow whole-body arousal. If arousal happens only from touching the clitoral crown, she may have a localized orgasm, which is more like a sneeze in intensity, bringing a simple relief of tension around the clitoris. With whole-body arousal, the orgasmic contractions emanate from the womb itself. With this intensity of release, there may be more contractions, or multiple orgasm – one orgasm leading directly into another and yet another, in one unbroken line. Another type of experience is chain orgasm, where one orgasm is very quickly followed by another. The orgasms are separate but they feed one into the next in quick succession, like the links in a chain.

Sometimes a woman may enjoy a slow delicious build-up into one tremendous climax. However, it is common for a woman to feel the need for between three and six orgasms in a single love session. The more orgasms a woman has, the stronger they become, and also, the more orgasms she has, the more she *can* have.

The varying moods of intensity in orgasm are all wonderful to explore. Through orgasm you can discover your vast capacity for ecstasy – for women, orgasmic capacity is seemingly limitless. After orgasm, the woman is left in the same type of space as during the pre-orgasmic build-up, often called the "after glow". This after glow remains for at least 20 minutes and it is good to celebrate it with "after-play" (see chapter 15).

the nectar of Amrita

Amrita, meaning nectar, is a jet or fine mist of fluid, that may be released during sex. It may soak a large area of the bed, or shoot as high as 6 feet (2m) into the air, but it is so light that it evaporates quickly. Some people call this female ejaculation. Women who have not been taught about it may mistake it for urine when it occurs, and be very embarrassed. In Tantric texts Amrita is prized as a regenerating substance. The man prided himself on his expertise as a lover if he could provoke this in a woman and was then able to drink its life-renewing nectar.

Physically, Amrita probably comes from the urethral sponge, also known as the G-spot (see page 23). There is a theory that this is the female version of the male prostate gland (which produces the fluid for semen). Since all embryos start with the same genital bulb, which then differentiates into either male or female structures, it seems possible that women may have a prostate-like gland. Chinese erotic texts call the G-spot area the "Palace of Yin" and describe it as the origin of the orgasmic "moon flower medicine". To locate the G-spot, the man can insert his ring finger into the Yoni and then slowly pull this finger back toward the opening, feeling along the front wall of the Yoni. The G-spot is a small area not far from the opening. It may feel a little rougher to the touch, and it may be slightly raised.

Amrita can be released before, during, or after orgasm. Emotionally it gives rise to a transcendental space beyond time and mind, which brings a religious quality to the experience. It usually occurs through deep penetration, when the woman is in a profound state of ecstatic let go. It can also happen through massage of the G-spot. However, it cannot usually be provoked through deliberate effort, but rather happens unpredictably and spontaneously when the woman is open and flowing with her sensual energy. Some women release Amrita quite often, while others do so rarely or not at all.

full-body orgasm

This may or may not include genital release and occurs when the erogenous zones all over the woman's body are activated and resonating like a finely tuned instrument. Instead of the erotic energy being focused on the clitoris, it is as if the clitoris has released its exquisite sensitivity all over the entire body. The whole of the woman, body and soul, becomes orgasmic. She may laugh, cry, scream, or howl from a space of delirious ecstasy.

This type of orgasmic experience is very close to spiritual awakening that Tantra considers it to be the portal of the goddess. When the woman passes this threshold she discovers her goddess nature, she who contains the whole universe, she who is the womb for all of life. The key to attaining this type of openness is through the awakening of the positive female centers (see chapter 8).

"Surrendering, relaxing, letting go
a very deep surrender to whatever.
Being a drop that falls into a river
Cascading, continually dropping deeper,
Knowing I am the drop
Yet I am dissolving in the river
Personal wants have gone"

Female Tantra group participant

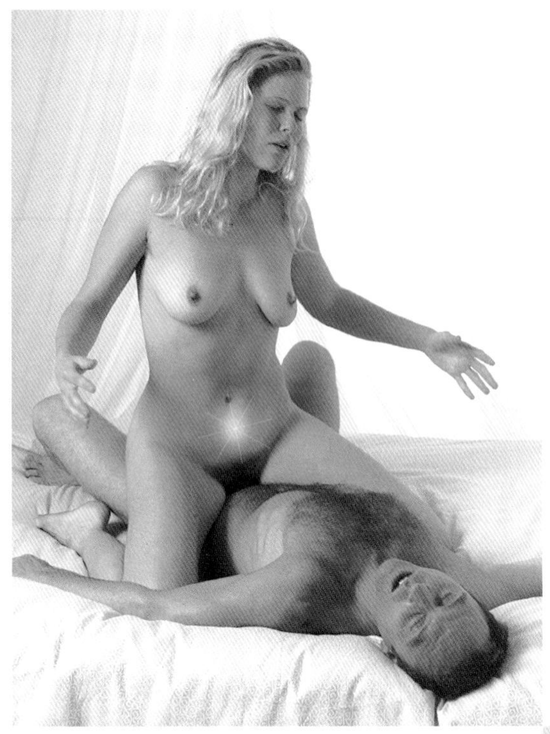

expanding orgasmic capacity

When you are self-pleasuring, or in the act of sex with a partner, you can expand your area of sensation to include your positive poles and then your whole body.

The captions below for the woman describe her focus during lovemaking; the captions for the man describe his focus (see pages 54–9) . You do not have to communicate verbally – just each be in your own flow, in a process of self-discovery and expansion.

♡ **Women** Imagine your belly expanding more and more, until you feel that you are simply a huge womb – the womb of the universe. Let sounds and emotions flow. Cry, laugh, sing – however you can best express this experience of vastness.

♡ **Men** When pleasure is triggered around the genitals, sense your Lingam as a wand of light, connected to universal life force energy.

♡ **Women** Bring your awareness to your heart center. Feel and visualize your breasts expanding. In your imagination, let that area of your body open like a flower, a magnificent flower in full bloom, full of fragrance. Express all the vast amount of love you have hidden inside, through sound, movement, and feeling. Allow yourself to experience orgasm from the heart.

♡ **Men** Shift your awareness and imagine that you are making love from the solar plexus; share your love and pleasure there for some time. Forget about your genitals. You may continue to move your body, but focus completely on the solar plexus and make love from there, as if penetrating her solar plexus on an energy level. The solar plexus (3rd chakra) is a positive pole in the man (see chapter 8). It is from there that he can communicate his strength and love.

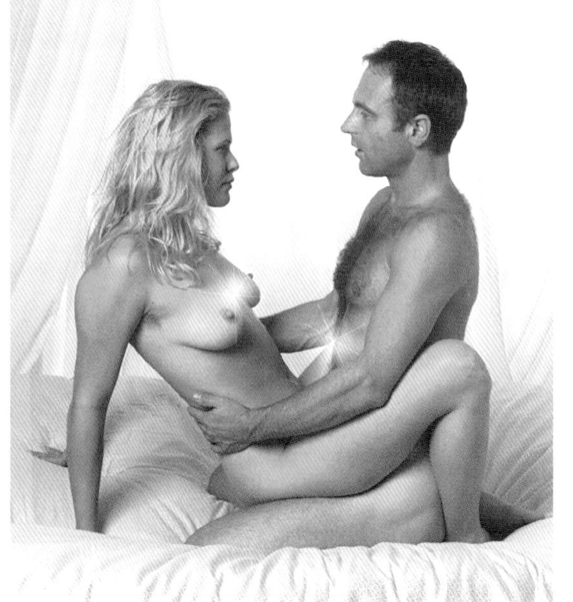

♡ **Women** Bring your awareness to your third eye center. Let this area be bathed with sensation, as if this is your Yoni in the act of love. You may experience tremendous inner light, or conversely, you may experience falling into deep velvety darkness without beginning or end.

♡ **Men** Next shift your awareness to the throat area (5th chakra). How would your love like to be expressed? Perhaps you would like to say sweet words of appreciation to your lover, or to make sounds. Allow your sexual energy and your love to be expressed through your sounds and language.

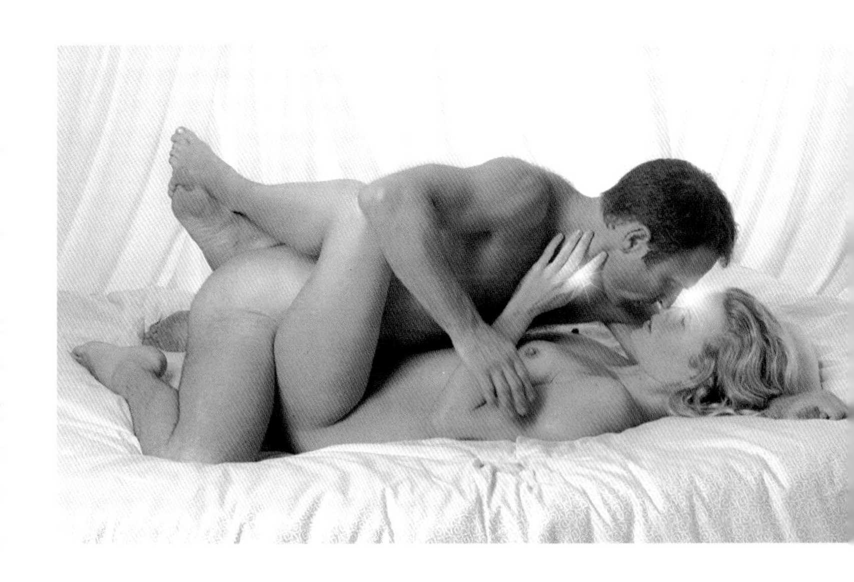

♡ **Both** Now you are ready to let go. Do not focus on any particular part of your body, but on yourself as a whole. Experience your whole body and energy at once – let go of the density of your body. Consider yourself as pure energy, moving your body or not, making sounds or not, just a play of energies taking you over. You are not doing, the energies are doing it for you and you just allow it to happen. The moment you are completely lost in the experience and the energy has taken over, you will know what Tantra is.

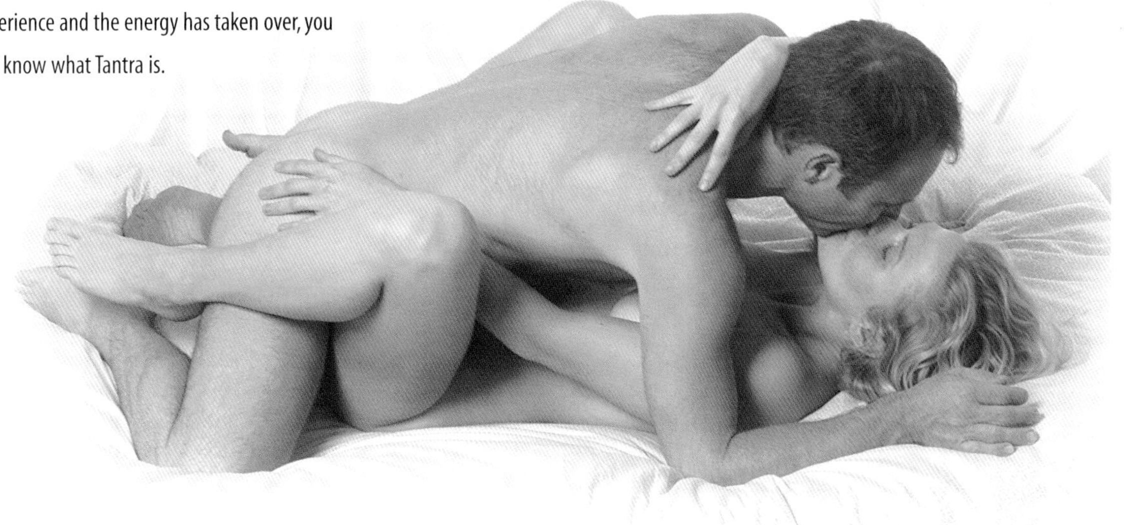

Male orgasm

"The popular term for sexual climax, 'coming' is such an interesting choice of word. Who is it that is arriving? Clearly the divinity in the man is arriving."

From *Manhood*, by Steve Biddulph

Male energy is often thought of as strong and rigid. But even though men often like to demonstrate their strength, a lot of the desire to prove it is simply a way of hiding their vulnerability. Male energy is actually more fragile than female energy. You can see this in the male body – the male genitals are "sticking out". The expression "sticking your neck out" means to put yourself in a vulnerable position. The position and form of the male genitals mean that a man is always in that position. He can't really hide.

It is usually obvious to others (especially women) when a man is trying to hide his vulnerability and sensitivity. If he can embrace his sensitive nature, he will feel more confident with himself. He does not become weak, but discovers a new and deeper strength he had not known before. A warrior is strong only if he is conscious of how vulnerable he is – only then can he act in full awareness. Otherwise the act of trying to prove his strength wastes his energy, making him weak.

In sex, the man who tries to hide his uncertainty and put on a "good performance" is often a bad lover, just as he would be a bad warrior, because he is not really connected to his own source of energy and power. This lack of connection means he is not fully connected to his partner either.

A man making love feels exposed, especially because he often believes that he has to have an erection throughout. If he tries to hide behind performance, or a mechanical way of lovemaking, his powerful Yang energy cannot emerge. However, when he stops trying to control the situation, he can be more relaxed and allow his Yang energy to flow. He drops the most difficult and tiring job on earth, of trying to prove himself. This gives him the freedom to be more connected to his energy and his partner's, enjoying the moment for what it is – a precious moment of pleasure and love flowing through his Lingam and every pore of his being.

This type of sensitivity transforms an ordinary man into a master lover, a god. In this state the man is open to the woman and actually receives energy from her. She will shower so much love and energy on him that the circle will be complete. You can go on making love like that for hours and you may not even care about ejaculation, because the lovemaking will be so rich, so full of delight. But even if you ejaculate, the exchange of energies will be so powerful that you will not feel you have lost energy – you will feel more full and satisfied.

The physiology of ejaculation

As the man becomes aroused, impulses pass through the sacral area to the Lingam. The arteries in the Lingam dilate, causing blood to fill the spongy areas in the shaft (see page 31). This raises the internal pressure and the Lingam becomes stiff and erect. If sexual arousal continues, which may involve physical stimulation directly on the shaft and tip of the Lingam as well as the whole genital area, the pressure mounts in intensity, reaching a plateau. The testicles engorge to 50 per cent larger than normal; breathing rate, heart rate, and blood pressure increase. These intense physical sensations are accompanied by waves of pleasure, which may create a sense of delirious cliff-hanging expectation that an explosion beyond mental control is about to happen.

There comes a point of no return, when impulses from the spinal cord at the level of the first and second lumbar vertebrae pass to muscles at the base of the Lingam, causing spasms that in turn bring about contractions in the seminal ducts (see page 31). These contractions send sperm into the urethra. Simultaneous contractions in the prostate gland and seminal vesicles expel prostate and seminal fluid to mix with the sperm. This mixture creates semen, a rich, slightly sticky white liquid. Rhythmic contractions originating in the first and second sacral vertebrae pass through muscles at the base of the Lingam and cause the semen to be ejaculated out from the urethra in from three to seven spurts, at intervals of 0.8 seconds.

This process of ejaculation is commonly called orgasm. The experience is controlled by an automatic (involuntary) reflex, which is beyond mental control, although the will can inhibit the orgasm reflex (see chapter 6). It is accompanied by sensations of intense pleasure, bringing a sense of deep let go, and a glimpse of infinity. This is why the experience of orgasm can be used as a jumping board into profoundly spiritual states of being.

"Being swept away, lifted, expanded

All of my pores opening

Spinning vortices of energy

Creamy delicious flying fire

Clouds of fire

The biggest 'yes' I can give

This side of death"

Male Tantra group participant

Releasing emotional energy

The way that life energy functions in the body is directly linked to sexuality. Life force energy, called Chi by the Chinese, Qi by the Japanese, and Prana in the Indian tradition, is all around us, omnipresent. A healthy child is a flowing, alive organism that attracts a sufficient amount of life force energy to function at an optimum. Unlike most adults, the child is a free-flowing being. He has access to so much energy that it is often too much for the adults. If the child is prevented from expressing this life force naturally, for example if he has to sit still for long periods in school and other similar situations, and is constantly controlled by adults (Don't do that; Don't be like this) he learns to "sit" on and suppress his bubbling life force. This life force, having no natural way of expression, accumulates around the liver and gall bladder. This store of energy constantly seeks expression and the child becomes fidgety.

If, as is so often the case in our "civilized" world, every day of his life he is prevented from living his spontaneous energy, this accumulated energy will be desperate for discharge. It may seek expression through a sudden burst of anger, as in a tantrum. Unfortunately that expression is usually not welcome either, so the child will have to repress that energy a little deeper. Sadness is the next one on the list of possibilities of expression. If the sadness is not really allowed (Don't be sad; Don't cry) then the same energy will have to be repressed a little deeper and turn into depression. Depression is usually allowed. If it becomes extreme the person will be put on medication to alleviate the symptoms. However, this doesn't find or cure the root cause and so is a poor solution. The boy will often be bored and unexcited about what life has to offer. He will have lost some of his spark, his natural sense of wonder.

Being unable to express your energy naturally is just about everyone's story, more or less. As an adult, the patterns you learned in childhood, of sitting on the natural expressions of your life force, are still there. But the life force goes on seeking expression. It has to get moving somehow, it is part of its nature to circulate, but energy is rarely allowed to move spontaneously.

That is why there is so much anger, irritability, stress, and depression all around. Many people cannot sit still for more than a few minutes in silence, because that repressed energy inside keeps them fidgety.

One easy way men have found to let go of the uncomfortable accumulated emotional charge is to ejaculate. The more unexpressed emotional energies or stagnant life force he has, the more the man will crave frequent ejaculation, just to get rid of that energy he no longer knows how to process naturally.

It is good to remember that such a pattern is not your fault; it will have originated in your emotional conditioning during childhood. The pattern of using sex for emotional release can be transformed through several ways: Primal therapy or other emotional release based therapies, bio-energetic therapy, Eriksonian hypnotherapy, color light therapy, and Tantra can all help in changing this habit. Experimenting with the methods we are proposing in this book will powerfully support you in embracing a healthy and uplifting sexual expression.

"Surging, burning joyful rising of energy

A sort of black out

I don't know where I am

Losing all sense of time and space

Just floating"

Male Tantra group participant

"The two of us become the universe

Like a vast night sky in the Sahara

So dark, with stars so bright

Becoming the cosmos"

Male Tantra group participant

"The sweetest, sweetest, sweetest

Melting of my prick and

Spreading further out through my body

A longing and loving feeling

Of sweet melting"

Male Tantra group participant

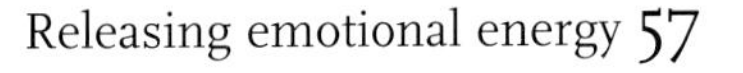

the four expressions of male sexual energy

1 the natural cycle of ejaculation

The body creates sperm and infuses it with a large quantity of vital energy taken from its own inner resources. Once ejaculated, that quantity of vital energy is lost forever. It is known in Tantra that a man has a certain number of ejaculations pre-programmed from birth. When a man uses ejaculation simply for emotional release, or as a sedative to have a good sleep afterward, he is stealing his own resources to do so. If he continues such practices for a long period, he may weaken his body and shorten his life span. It is wise to discover your own natural cycle for ejaculatory pleasure, rather than wasting the life force by using ejaculation to release pent-up emotional and mental tension.

When a couple follows Tantra teachings, their lovemaking becomes richer in many dimensions. Their energies start to merge and recharge each other. Those experiences are so fulfilling that genital orgasm becomes much less of a focus. The man's body can then come to a more natural cycle of ejaculation. The frequency and physical need for ejaculation is individual, and depends upon the man's age, state of health, and genetic disposition.

It is possible for a man to recuperate and recharge the energy he has lost in previous ejaculations. Lovemaking without ejaculation, where the man and the woman experience a deep union in the merging of at least three chakras (see pages 52–3), is a way to recharge and reverses the loss of vital energy due to past ejaculations.

2 opening the channel, redirecting the energy

In the body, vital energy can move upward or downward. The downward movement is the most common – it just follows the intent that nature has programmed. In sex the energy gets triggered and accumulates in the pelvic area. This build-up comes to a climax and comes down and out though ejaculation of semen.

Energy always follows intent. With the downward movement of energy, nature's intent is procreation and continuation of the species. The upward movement of energy is also created through intent, but this time, it comes through a conscious decision to expand into new realms of being. Moving upward is another expression of sexual energy, which opens up new possibilities and experiences.

The exercise "Expanding orgasmic capacity" on page 52 will help you to experience the redirecting and expansion of orgasmic energy. If you are without a sexual partner and wish to experiment with this, you can use the "Love yourself as a man" exercise (see pages 46–7).

3 conserving semen

In Tantra you can learn to conserve semen, which allows the body energy to go on increasing and expanding, helping the bodily functions to move to a greater state of health and vitality. The increase of energy also provokes an awakening and heightening of the senses, bringing in new types of pleasure and satisfaction as a reward. Ultimately this practice opens up to a new possibility of whole-body orgasm.

Conserving semen or "retention of ejaculation" is often believed to require effort and control. On the contrary, the art of conserving semen involves love, relaxation, and let go. This let go, coupled with awareness and intent to invite sexual energy to move upward and reunite with the systems in the brain (see chapter 3), leads to a state that can be called "becoming orgasmic".

Occasional retention of ejaculation is good practice and can be experimented with freely. However, if you intend to go through a series of Tantric practice without ejaculating for more than three times in a row, your body has to be in good basic health. When your body is overloaded, it uses semen to expel the excess toxins it cannot get rid of by other means. If you do not ejaculate, these toxins are then reabsorbed into your body. In ancient India and China, where Tantra was developed, health was always a priority as an integral part of the practice. Adepts used Ayurveda and Yoga in India, and Chi Kung, acupuncture, and herbs in China to detox. Before starting to practice conserving semen, you should first undertake a full-body detox, over a period of about three months, using herbs, plants, and plant extracts (see Resources, page 188).

The prostate gland plays an important role in the conservation of semen, as it is there that the non-ejaculated energy builds up. The practice can cause some tension in the prostate, resulting in a dull ache all around the genitals. Most men know this aching, if they have made love without coming. However this aching usually goes after three or four non-ejaculatory lovemaking sessions. If it is still present after four or five love sessions, it is better to ejaculate and discontinue the conservation of semen process.

Some Chinese-style methods suggest rhythmically contracting the pelvic muscles to help release tension in the prostate gland, thus recycling the precious prostate fluid back into the system for health and longevity. However, the body will reabsorb the sperm and prostate fluid anyway, and rhythmic pumping of the pelvic muscles may create tension in the pelvic floor, inhibiting proper grounding. It may also affect the subtle energy connection between head and pelvis, which is important for spiritual development (see chapter 3).

Conserving semen is best practiced in conjunction with step two, opening the pathways to channel energy toward higher states of love and consciousness. Without Tantric methods to support the process, it is difficult to experience the full benefit of the practice.

4 becoming orgasmic

Becoming orgasmic is the highest potential of sexual energy. In this state, sexual energy is recycled back to its origin in the brain, infusing the whole body with an ecstasy far beyond the normal experience of orgasm. It is a reunion with the whole, a floating in space beyond time and mind. Sometimes you reach this state spontaneously during lovemaking. When it takes them by surprise, the couple may wait for years or a lifetime, hoping that it will happen again.

The fact that it happens spontaneously to some people shows that this state is natural and accessible to everyone. The ancient Tantra masters devised methods to make exalted union available to anyone who is willing to learn. The exercises in this book use some of these methods, including breathing exercises, meditation, and touch, opening the five senses, and Tantric sexual intercourse.

creating an orgasmic lifestyle for men and women

♡ Take pen and paper. Close your eyes and write about what happens to you in the moment of orgasm. Use your left hand if you are right-handed, and vice versa. Let your writing be a "stream of consciousness". Don't allow your conscious mind to interfere with the act of writing, just let go and allow it to happen spontaneously.

♡ Read over your writing and pick out the key words that you can apply in your daily life. For example, the states of let go, love, bliss, expansion, being present in this moment, melting in the universe, are all highly prized spiritual states. If you apply these qualities to relating, or drinking tea, or eating, or exercising, or working, you will transform your own life and the lives of those around you. The spiritual teachings of all the mystics through the ages are contained as a blueprint in your own orgasmic capacity. Learn from your own body and apply this teaching to your life.

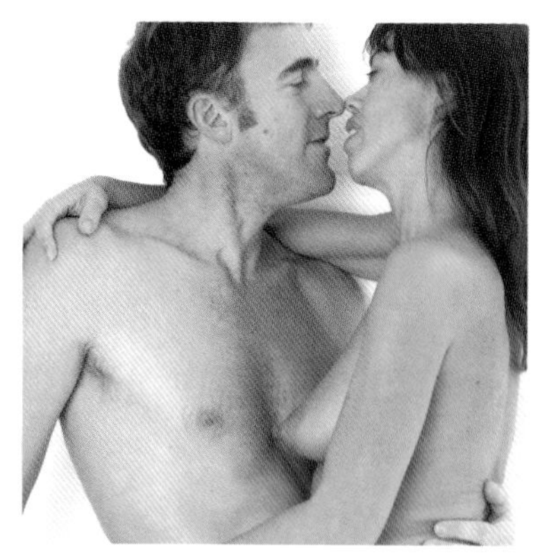

physical mechanics of the sex act

"If anyone asks you how the perfect satisfaction
of all our sexual wanting
will look, lift your face and say,
'Like this'."
Jelaluddin Rumi, Sufi mystic, translated by Coleman Barks

Sex is the most powerful force on earth: the force that generates life in all its myriad forms. Since we owe our lives to the sex act, it is worthy of our reverence and deserves respectful attention.

As human beings we need to ask ourselves, "What is sex? How can we best experience it? How can we learn from it for our highest evolution?" If we do not have role models who are living the answers to these questions, it is more difficult for us to find our way. Human happiness and a harmonious society depend on those answers. And yet we keep pushing the subject under the carpet, or perverting it, or pretending to know all about it while remaining confused inside.

"The whole universe from Brahman to the smallest worm is based on the union of male and female."

Vrihat Samhita (Indian scripture)

Learning about sex

The way people learn about sex is often a sad commentary on how our society "deals with" sex. Our experience of working in Tantra groups and holistic healing sessions, and finding out how much suffering is related to misinformed ideas about sex, encouraged us to write this book. Many people with apparently normal lives are in deep anguish, because they do not know a few very simple sexual guidelines. This is not their fault. A large part of human education takes place through example. People are usually raised in nuclear families, sex is not discussed, the parents may fight, demonstrations of affection may be rare, and there may even be violence. Sex takes place furtively, shamefully, and in hiding. A child may overhear muffled sexual sounds, which are often interpreted as the mother being tortured.

Let us compare the human experience with Bonobos, a type of ape and the animals closest to humans in terms of their sexual nature. A Bonobo tribe has no leader and no hierarchy; there is no violence or war. Like humans, Bonobos are able to become aroused at any time. As a tribe, they often get sexually aroused before eating, and then enjoy an orgy of copulation as "hors d'oeuvres". They have no hierarchy or preference for who they mate with. Old mix with young easily and naturally. Adult males and females enjoy screaming orgasms. They have sex in varied positions. Before they reach sexual maturity the young imitate these activities as a form of play. We are not suggesting that humans should behave like Bonobos. However, we can see from their example that when sex is learned and celebrated in a playful and natural way, this contributes to a non-violent society.

The physical act

In sex, opposites attract. Male and female are opposite and complementary in their bodies, psyches, and subtle energetic systems. The male Lingam is a positive pole, with an outward or Yang energy. When the man is sexually aroused, his Lingam signals that he is ready for sexual pleasure by becoming erect. It may pulsate with life energy and secrete a milky liquid. This is accompanied by a longing for penetration.

The female Yoni is a receptive pole, with an inward or Yin energy. When the woman is sexually aroused, her breasts may swell and her nipples may become erect. Her vagina enlarges and lengthens in a type of internal erection, just the size needed to fit snugly around her partner's Lingam. Her clitoris may swell and come out of hiding. Her vagina may secrete copious amounts of liquid and she may feel a deep longing to touch her clitoris and to be penetrated inside her vagina.

Pre-orgasmic build-up generally takes a longer time for the woman than it does for the man. To come to full arousal, the woman needs her positive energy poles stimulated, in her belly, breasts, and third eye (see chapter 8). Once these are awakened her receptive energy poles, including her Yoni, will function fully. Therefore the man and woman need to learn a balance in how they initiate love play (see chapter 15).

When a man and woman come close to each other in this state of pre-orgasmic build-up, they may feel something like an electric current passing between them, which makes them almost delirious with longing. Consummation can be in many

The way people learn about sex is too often a sad commentary on how sex is dealt with in our society. Some common examples are:

"I learned about it from things kids were saying in the school yard."

"I learned it in biology but couldn't understand anything from all those diagrams with Latin names. It was meaningless in terms of real human contact."

"I heard about it in the Sunday school when the nun told us we would go to hell for it."

"My mother told me while we were driving in the car, but she seemed so uptight that I just felt sick and disgusted and couldn't wait to get out of the car."

"I saw porno movies with my friend that we had sneaked from his Dad."

"I lived on a farm so I saw the animals doing it."

ways: kissing the lips and the whole body, merging tongues, sucking nipples, caressing the whole body, kissing, caressing, and smelling each other's genitals, and penetrative sex. For penetration the man and woman join their pelvises so that the man's Lingam can enter the woman's Yoni. When these two opposite and complementary poles meet, it often creates such a sense of wellbeing and nurturing that the couple would like to remain in that state forever. However nature, seeking the procreation of the species, urges the couple to make movements that maximize genital pleasure, driving them toward genital release through orgasm. The couple trained in the arts of love knows how to outwit nature's procreative aspect and maximize pleasure for hours without necessarily seeking genital release. An untrained couple may find themselves fumbling heatedly for a short time, moving into penetrative sex and orgasmic release for one or both partners within a period of a few minutes.

At orgasm the man ejaculates. His semen carries a vibration of his mental and emotional state. Women are sensitive to this: receiving semen in the Yoni is drinking in the man's essence. If this essence is charged with negative emotion it may feel repugnant to the woman, but if it is charged with love the woman will feel she has received a benediction that nourishes her very being.

After ejaculation the man's Lingam becomes soft and flaccid. He may feel a sudden loss of energy and wish to sleep or rest. Nature invests a lot of energy in the continuation of the species, and the man donates a little of his life force to this purpose every time he ejaculates. A wise man will not ejaculate every time, but will learn how to savor the delights of love while saving the release of sperm for special occasions.

Self-image

Self-image is an important factor in sexuality. Many men worry about the size of their genitals, while many women worry about being too fat or too thin, about the appearance of their genitals, or the shape and size of their breasts.

From their school days, boys tend to compare the size of their penises with others. Men have always been preoccupied with penis size: Vatsyayana's *Kama Sutra*, from the 4th century,

male sexual dysfunction

There are three common possibilities:

1) Inability to experience erection, called erectile dysfunction or impotence.

2) Premature ejaculation.

3) Inability to ejaculate, called ejaculatory incompetence or retarded ejaculation.

According to Tantra, these problems all have their root in the stagnation of energy flow in one or more areas of the body. The following techniques promote free energy flow.

♡ Learn how to develop relaxed whole-body sensitivity, as in the caressing meditation (see page 157).

♡ Free yourself from psychological burdens and conditioning by allowing the circulation of breath and emotions (see pages 175–7). Other treatments that may be helpful include psychotherapy to encourage emotional release, acupuncture and Traditional Chinese Medicine, breath therapy (such as bio-energetics, rebirthing), craniosacral therapy, color light therapy, or bodywork.

♡ For premature ejaculation, learn how to take more time with sensual play. You can use self-pleasuring to start with, making it a meditation (see chapter 4). You may also find sessions with a sex therapist helpful.

♡ Inability to have an erection can be caused by many factors, including poor health, medication, surgical removal of the prostate, or excessive beer drinking (the hops in beer can cause impotence if taken in excess). Some medication can also cause erectile dysfunction; you should discuss this with your medical practitioner.

♡ In most cases, releasing emotional stagnation, eating a balanced diet, and taking regular exercise will improve any of these three conditions. Natural herbal remedies may also be effective.

♡ Most importantly, don't keep it a secret and suffer in silence. Seek qualified help and in most cases there will be dramatic improvement.

female sexual dysfunction

There are four common possibilities.

1) Inability to reach orgasm (even while self-pleasuring,) commonly called frigidity.

2) Non-arousal.

3) Inability to orgasm while making love with a man.

4) Inability to tolerate penetration to the extent that the Yoni is completely contracted, so that even insertion of a finger causes intense pain . This condition is called vaginismus.

Many women think they have sexual dysfunction when actually there is nothing wrong with them. They may have high expectations of how a woman should be during sex, which may have come from highly unrealistic literature or from the erroneous theory of vaginal versus clitoral orgasm (see page 49). If a woman is able to orgasm while self-pleasuring there is nothing wrong with her. All the joys of sex can emerge for her, if her feminine nature is allowed to flower.

♡ Inability to orgasm at all is usually rooted in psychological wounding or sexual abuse. Psychotherapy that allows and facilitates emotional release, hypnosis, and holistic healing methods such as color light therapy and craniosacral therapy can help dramatically with these issues.

♡ Non-arousal may be due to poor health, oral contraceptives (which can lower libido), or changes due to ageing. Natural herbal remedies to balance the hormonal system should bring positive results (see Resources, page 188).

♡ Vaginismus may be helped by sex therapy with a partner. First you need to allow your whole body to become more sensitive, as with the caressing meditation (see page 157). With the support of a sex therapist, you can follow this slowly, one step at a time, introducing a little finger into the opening, gradually increasing the depth of insertion, then a larger finger, and finally the Lingam. This process may take weeks, so a lot of patience and love is needed.

describes methods for enlarging the penis. However, for every size of Lingam there is a Yoni to fit it. Usually, if a man's energy is alive and flowing and he is relaxed around his sexual expression, women will be very happy with his size. It is not the size of your penis, but how relaxed, open, and fluid you are with your whole body and emotions that makes a good lover.

A woman who compares her breast size and shape to other women may imagine that larger breasts will bring her greater happiness. Many women now have breast implants, which may be damaging to their health and which destroy the breasts' natural sensitivity. A woman's breast size and sensitivity can be greatly enhanced through Tantric meditations and regular breast massage (see chapter 9). For tips and exercises on loving your own body, see chapter 1.

The divine nature of sex

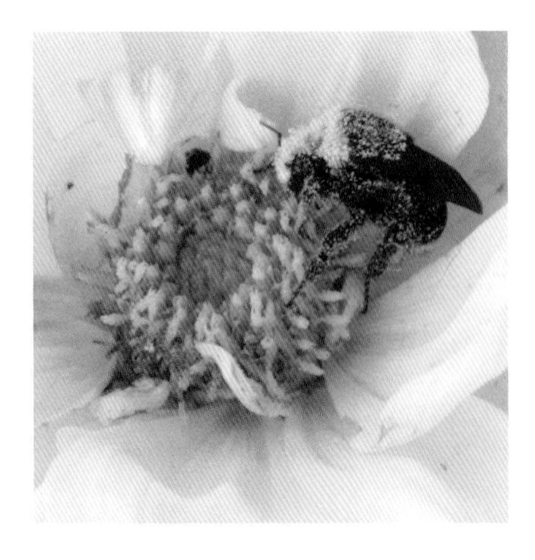

The sex act is key to all aspects of nature. Every time a bee takes nectar from a flower, it is a sexual act. The bee is ensuring not only its own survival but the survival of the plant, by spreading pollen between male and female plants. Fall in tune with a bee as it gathers nectar from a flower. Close your eyes and pretend you are that bee; feel what it feels – pure ecstasy, pure orgasm.

The meeting of heaven and earth is also a sexual dance. It is the energy of the masculine sun penetrating the atmosphere surrounding the feminine earth that creates the conditions conducive to life. In each aspect of creation we can see the act of sex and also feel the presence of the divine within it. The symmetry and harmony of nature give rise to feelings of awe and reverence, and at the same time we can see how the divine breathes life into being through the act of sex, through the meeting of the opposite poles of Yin and Yang. This is why many ancient societies have honoured the sex act so highly and made it a key part of acts of worship. It is through the intelligent study of sex that we can finally understand and embrace divinity.

Sex can lead you, if you allow it, into deep communion with your own soul and with the soul of the whole planet. In it is hidden the secret of the creation principle, which when understood unleashes genius, sensitivity, and love for all living beings.

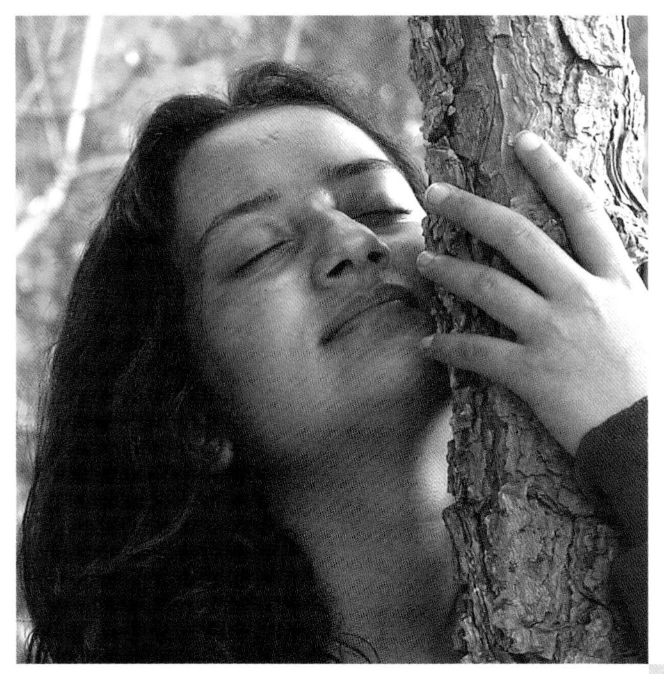

See the birds in their mating dance, the wonder of a peacock's tail, designed by nature to dazzle and hypnotize the female into compliance for the sex act. Watch cats stalking through the grass, the female lying coquettishly on her back as she lures the tomcat, then with what glee she jumps up and runs just out of reach as he comes close.

See the stallion, so fierce and proud, as he rears up on his hind legs beginning his courtship of the mare. Watch him as he becomes the most docile of suitors, nibbling her neck, nuzzling her flank, kissing her lips, and finally mounting her.

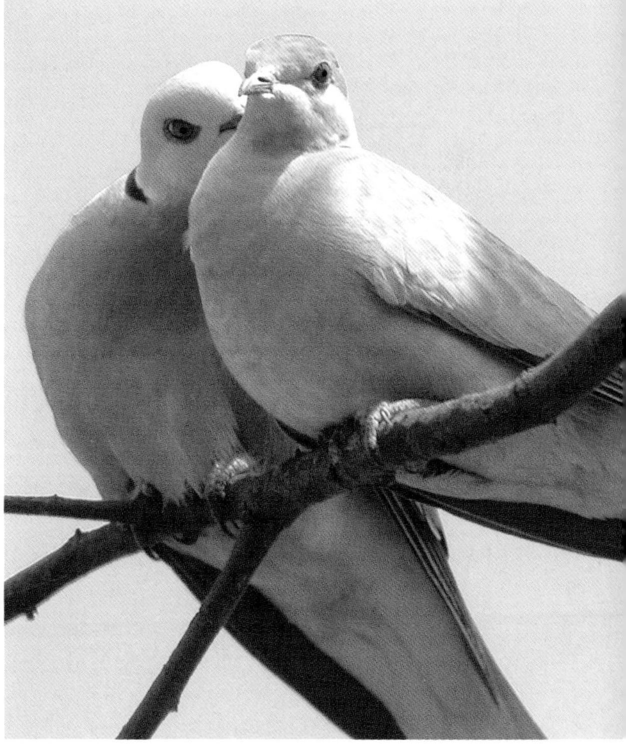

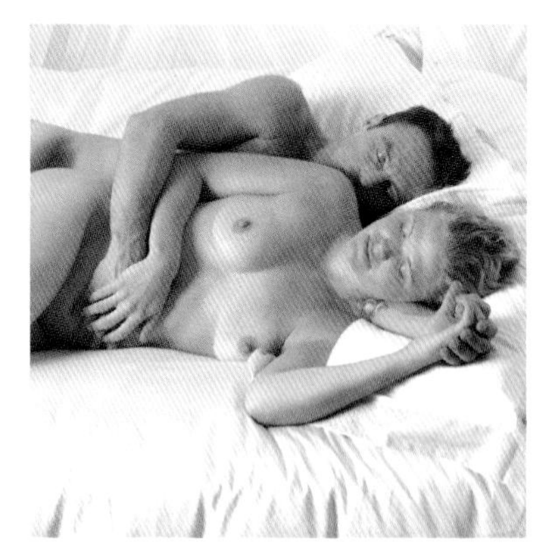

conception, birth control, and safe sex

"Make love a priority in your life
And everything you do will be for the best.
Love makes the universe turn
If we but know it
The intelligence of love
Is as supreme as it is subtle"
Jelaluddin Rumi, Sufi mystic, translated by Camille and Kabir Helminski

Conception

Centuries of Tantra research have shown that a couple's state of mind and the astrological configuration at the time of conception, as well as the physical attributes of the couple, all play an important role in forming the child. Your cells carry the memory of how your parents were thinking and feeling while they were conceiving you, and this first imprint is the foundation for how you experience life. Because of this, Tantricas approach the act of conception with great reverence and awareness.

The physical mechanics of conception

At ejaculation, the 300–500 million sperms carried in the semen travel up the woman's Yoni toward the womb. Spasmodic waves emanating deep inside her Yoni help them on their journey. If the woman is in her fertile phase (see page 89), her cervix will be producing a lot of slippery mucus to help the sperm reach the womb. More spasmodic waves from the walls of the womb then carry the sperm up into the fallopian tubes, in search of an egg cell to fertilize. Less than one per cent of sperm complete this long journey, and for conception usually only one sperm will penetrate the egg.

Fertilization, when the egg and sperm meet, may occur up to 24 hours after ejaculation. Once the egg is fertilized it travels to the womb, where it embeds in the womb lining and begins its nine-month gestation.

The Tantra approach

Conception is the invitation for a new life to come into being – a very auspicious moment. If you bring the light of awareness and love to this occasion, you send out an invitation to a soul who is in tune with these qualities to come to you. A soul is attracted into a physical body through two dimensions. One dimension is that soul's own development, or the karmic blueprint. Karma means in essence, "You reap what you sow." If a person dies with incomplete emotional issues, that unfinished business will seek completion by bringing the soul back for another round of birth and death. The karmic resonance between the parents and the soul coming to them helps to form the new life. In addition, a soul is attracted to the genetic structure that will best serve his or her karmic purpose.

In ancient Tantra societies, people were very aware that the type of soul coming to the earth plane is dependent on the level of consciousness of the couple at the moment of conception. Astrologers were consulted about the most auspicious time to conceive. The original Indian form of astrology uses the time of conception, not the time of birth, as the main reference point for making a chart. Couples would also consult a Guru, who would counsel them on how to create the most desirable ambience and on the type of lovemaking conducive to inviting a soul of great potential. It is said in Tantric scriptures that whatever type of being the woman fantasizes about while making love, this is the type of child who will be born to her. It was also thought that the type of food the woman ate before conception would influence the type of soul that would be attracted. And after conception and throughout the pregnancy, the woman was urged to maintain a state of sublime, loving calm, in order not to traumatize the delicate new life.

The choice to create and nurture a new life is a profound commitment, not to be made carelessly. Preparation and learning are needed before embarking on the journey. By approaching conception with reverence and awareness, we will ensure that physically and spiritually refined qualities become predominant in humankind.

"Only through sexual union are new beings capable of existing. This union, therefore, represents a place between two worlds, a point of contact between being and nonbeing; where life manifests itself and incarnates the divine spirit. The forms of the organs that achieve this ritual are symbolic. They are the visible form of the creator."

from *The Phallus*, by Alain Danielou

Birth control

To enjoy sexual freedom and to be able to make an intelligent choice of when to conceive, it is important to know how to prevent conception. Each birth control method has its pros and cons. Some of the most widely used methods are described below.

method	pros	cons
Rhythm and symto-thermal method The woman records her temperature regularly and observes other signs, such as changes in the vaginal mucus, to determine when she is fertile. During the fertile phase, you can avoid penetrative sex or use a barrier method (see below).	It is very freeing for a woman to be in tune with her own body. The fertile phase, when the egg is released from the ovary, generally occurs in a regular cycle over a 3–5 day period every month. The egg can only be fertilized during a 24-hour period in that time, but to be on the safe side you need to be careful 2–3 days before and after that 24-hour period.	The fertile phase is exactly when women long for very passionate sex, so you may "slip up" and find yourself pregnant. The method only suits women who have a very regular menstrual cycle. Also, some women ovulate on demand, so that even when they are supposedly not fertile, a passionate love session can stimulate the release of an egg.
Contraceptive sponge Barrier method: made of polyurethane and containing spermicide. It is inserted into the vagina to fit over the cervix, shortly before penetrative sex.	It is sold over the counter in some countries, and is as effective as the Diaphragm. It has been proven to reduce the risk of catching Gonorrhoea or Chlamydia.	It has been shown to increase the risk of vaginal infections caused by Candida. Some women are allergic to the spermicide. It has to be left in place for at least 6 hours after having sex.
Diaphragm Barrier method: a rubber dome that fits over the cervix. It needs to be filled with spermicide and inserted before penetrative sex. It then can be left in the vagina for up to 24 hours	If you know you have a hot date, you can insert it in advance. It may protect against some sexually transmitted infections.	The spermicide tastes terrible, so kissing the Yoni loses its charm. During deep penetration the Diaphragm can slip from its position. Some women are allergic to some spermicides. You have to keep it in for at least 6 hours after lovemaking. You will need a fitting with a doctor to determine the correct size for you.
Cervical cap Barrier method: a small thimble-shaped latex or silicone cap that fits snugly over the cervix. Generally used with spermicide, though there is a "honey cap", made of rubber which absorbs honey – a natural spermicide.	Smaller than the Diaphragm, and easier to insert. The honey cap is specially designed to be soaked in honey (don't try it with a normal cap) and rinsed off before insertion. The honey makes oral sex very sweet.	The suction can become uncomfortable. You have to keep it in for 6 hours after lovemaking. It can be knocked loose with deep penetration and you may need to check it during lovemaking. Some women are allergic to some spermicides. The spermicide makes the Yoni taste terrible. It has to be fitted by a doctor.

method	pros	cons
Male Condom Barrier method, made of non-porous latex or polyurethane and treated with spermicide. It is fitted snugly over the erect Lingam before penetration. At ejaculation, the semen is held inside the tip of the condom.	The man can take responsibility for birth control. It can be bought over the counter. It can prevent the transmission of sexually transmitted diseases, including HIV. As it is put on just prior to penetration, it is a good method to use in spontaneous sex.	Many men complain that it takes away a great deal of pleasurable sensation. Some men are not able to maintain erection while putting it on. With deep and forceful thrusting the condom may break. The Lingam has to withdraw from the Yoni almost immediately after ejaculation, so that the condom does not fall off and leak its contents into the Yoni. Some women are allergic to latex and some spermicides.
Female Condom A soft polyurethane sheath that lines the Yoni and covers the area just outside.	Can be put in any time before sex. It may protect both partners from sexually transmitted infections. Good to use if the man has problems with a male condom.	It may slip. Need to make sure the Lingam enters the condom, and not between the Yoni and the condom. Can make unpleasant noises during active penetration.
Intrauterine Device (IUD) A small device made of plastic, copper, or stainless steel, which is inserted into the womb. It prevents a fertilized egg embedding in the womb. It has a small plastic string that hangs out of the cervix into the vagina.	Once it has been fitted, it can remain in place for 3–10 years, but it can be taken out (by a doctor) at any time.	There may be a nagging sensation in the womb, producing tension in one of the main female positive poles and preventing the woman from feeling open during sex. During penetration contact between the Lingam and the plastic string may cause cramping sensations in the woman. It has to be fitted by a doctor. It can make menstruation heavier and may increase the risk of pelvic inflammatory disease.
Intrauterine System (IUS) A small plastic device that releases the hormone progestogen. It is inserted in the womb, like an IUD. It thickens the cervical mucus to stop sperm meeting an egg, and may also stop an egg implanting in the womb, or stop ovulation.	Once it has been fitted, it can remain in place for 5 years, but it can be taken out (by a doctor) at any time. Menstruation will usually be lighter.	Irregular bleeding is common for the first three months, and perhaps longer. Side effects may include headaches, acne, and tender breasts. It can make menstruation more prolonged and irreguar, and may increase the risk of pelvic inflammatory disease.

method	pros	cons
Combined pill A synthetic hormone compound of progesterone and estrogen, which stops ovulation by tricking the body into thinking it is already pregnant. It is taken in a regular 28-day cycle, starting on day 1 of menstruation. From day 27 to day 5 of the next cycle there are no pills, or pills with no hormones, to allow bleeding.	Over 99% effective in preventing pregnancy if taken as prescribed. Often reduces menstrual bleeding and period pain.	Commonly reported side effects include bloating and weight gain, spider veins, varicose veins, nausea, headaches, increase in facial hair, breakthrough bleeding between periods, and loss of sexual desire. In some women it may increase the risk of thrombosis, breast and cervical cancer. It is prescribed by a doctor and you will need regular check-ups. Its effectiveness is reduced if you have a stomach upset, or take other medication, e.g. antibiotics, or are more than 12 hours late taking it.
Progestogen-only pill The hormone progestogen thickens cervical mucus to prevent sperm meeting an egg, or to prevent an egg embedding in the womb. In some women it prevents ovulation.	It has fewer reported side effects than the combined pill and it is 99% effective if taken according to instructions.	It has to be taken at exactly the same time each day to be effective. Vomiting, diarrhoea, and some medications may reduce its effectiveness, but it is not affected by antibiotics. Periods may be irregular; there may be some spotting. Possible side effects include breast discomfort and increased risk of ovarian cysts.
Contraceptive injection An injection into the buttocks or arm muscle every 2–3 months, which releases progestogen slowly into the body. This stops ovulation and thickens cervical mucus, preventing sperm from reaching an egg.	Almost 100% effective. Allows for trouble-free sex since you don't have to worry about taking a pill every day or using a barrier method.	You cannot change your mind once you have had the injection. You may not be able to become pregnant for up to 2 years after an injection. Possible side effects include weight gain, loss of libido, vaginal dryness, risk of arterial disease, and osteoporosis. Most women either stop menstruating or have irregular spotting. Some women have prolonged and heavy bleeding.
Hormonal implants A small plastic tube inserted under the skin of the upper arm under local anaesthetic. It releases progestogen into the body, to stop ovulation and thicken cervical mucus, preventing sperm from reaching an egg.	Works for up to 3 years, but can be removed (by a doctor) at any time. When it is removed your normal level of fertility should return immediately.	The implant may cause localized pain, swelling, and infection of the arm. Menstruation may be much heavier, irregular, or stop altogether. Other side effects may include headaches, acne, tender breasts, nausea, mood swings, weight gain or loss, and increased risk of ovarian cysts.

method	pros	cons
Withdrawal Generally used if no other method is available. Just prior to ejaculation the man withdraws his Lingam from the Yoni.	It reduces the risk of conception.	The man may not manage to withdraw before ejaculating. Some sperm may leak out through the urethra prior to full ejaculation. Anxiety creates tension in both partners, inhibiting pleasure.
PERMANENT METHODS **Female sterilization** A surgical method under full anaesthetic. An incision is made in the belly and the fallopian tubes are tied and cut. Healing may take up to ten days. It is more complex surgery than male sterilization.	Permanent birth control, with no known long-term side effects.	Some women experience tension or pain in the area. Very rarely the fallopian tubes rejoin and the woman is fertile again. The operation cannot always be reversed successfully if you change your mind and wish to become pregnant.
Male sterilization/ vasectomy Simple surgery under local anaesthetic. An incision is made on either side of the scrotum and the tubes that carry the sperm are cut. The incision heals within a few days.	Permanent birth control with no discernible side effects. At orgasm the man ejaculates semen and the sperm is reabsorbed into the body. For a man who does not want to father more children, it is by far the best contraceptive method.	If you change your mind later and decide you wish to father a child, it may not be possible to reverse the surgery effectively. Very rarely the tubes may rejoin so the man is fertile again.
EMERGENCY METHODS **Emergency Pill** A pill containing synthetic hormones, that may prevent or delay ovulation, or stop a fertilized egg implanting in the womb. In some countries it is available over the counter, in others you will need to see a doctor.	It can be taken up to 72 hours after sex, but is most effective if taken in the first 24 hours.	Side effects can include nausea, vomiting, headaches, dizziness, and abdominal pain. It may cause irregular bleeding before your next menstrual period. It is not recommended for frequent use as it disrupts your menstrual cycle.
Intrauterine Device (IUD) Insertion of an IUD up to 5 days after unprotected sex prevents fertilization, or prevents a fertilized egg implanting in the womb.	The most effective emergency method. If you do not want to use the IUD as an ongoing method of contraception, it can be removed once you are sure you are not pregnant.	As for the IUD (see page 69). You have to have it fitted by a nurse or doctor, and you will need a follow-up appointment later either to check it is still in place, or to have it removed.

Safe sex

Safe sex means sex practiced in such a way that neither you or your partner are at risk of contaminating each other with one of over two dozen sexually transmitted diseases.

Before the discovery of penicillin, Syphilis and Gonorrhoea led to physical and mental degeneration and death. This is one reason for the many Victorian taboos around sexuality. These diseases are still around but can now be treated effectively with antibiotics. However, other sexually transmitted diseases cannot yet be cured. HIV infection may lead to full-blown AIDS. Herpes is not fatal, but can be extremely painful, and since a woman risks transmitting it to her baby at birth, she may be expected to have a caesarian section rather than giving birth normally.

Lovers everywhere need to face up to the fact that unless both partners have been tested for sexually transmitted diseases, including HIV, and are all clear, it is not safe to make love without using condoms. For many sexually transmitted diseases, you can be a carrier without experiencing any of the symptoms of the disease. Ideally, both partners should take responsibility for practicing safe sex. With a monogamous relationship it makes sense for you both to go for a medical check before you start practising sex without condoms. It is also essential to have honest communication between lovers, and to tell each other if one of you has a new sexual partner.

If you have multiple partners you will need to use condoms every time. Medical checks cannot work on a daily or weekly basis: if a person has become infected with HIV this may not show in medical tests for several months.

Many men are very reluctant to use condoms, but it is no use berating them about it. A woman simply has to learn to be creative and firm, bringing her qualities of love, understanding, and compassion to create a truly fun condom experience.

"We used to live in a community of about 5000 people, where free-flowing sexual expression was the norm. When AIDS became an issue, everyone was asked to use condoms and have regular tests for sexually transmitted disease every 3 months. Naturally, we became very inventive in the use of condoms, taking it as a matter of pride to be able to have marvellous sex while using them.

I had several lovers in those days, since I was into exploring all the different facets of my sexuality. When a lover came to my house, we would perhaps share a bath or a massage. Then I would put on some music and bring a tray of tea, decorated with flowers and a selection of condoms. When we were making love, and it was clear that the moment had come for penetration, I would unwrap the condom, and deftly guide it over my lover's erect Lingam. After ejaculation, when I felt the Lingam beginning to shrink, he would withdraw and one of us would remove the condom. I would then go to the bathroom, and wash (see page 73). Then I would wet a soft washcloth, which I called a love towel, with steaming hot water and carry it back to my lover. I would wash his Lingam with great care, and then dry it with another soft love towel. This whole procedure was so nourishing that I think none of my lovers ever felt in the least bit dissatisfied with the use of the condom."

Sarita

"It is love that makes sex special. Any act done with love is transformed into something divine – even putting on a condom."

sexual hygiene

The simple act of washing the genital area straight after lovemaking does not prevent pregnancy or serious diseases, but it can help to prevent Candida and urinary tract infections.

Add 2 teaspoons of cider vinegar to a mug of warm water and wash as described below.

♡ For the woman, wash inside and all around the Yoni using the fingers. An easy way to do this is to squat down in the shower, with your legs apart. You can then rinse with clear water. Washing with the fingers is gentle and does not disturb the Yoni's natural flora, or its lubricating and self-cleansing capacity.

♡ For the man, wash the Lingam carefully, pulling back the foreskin.

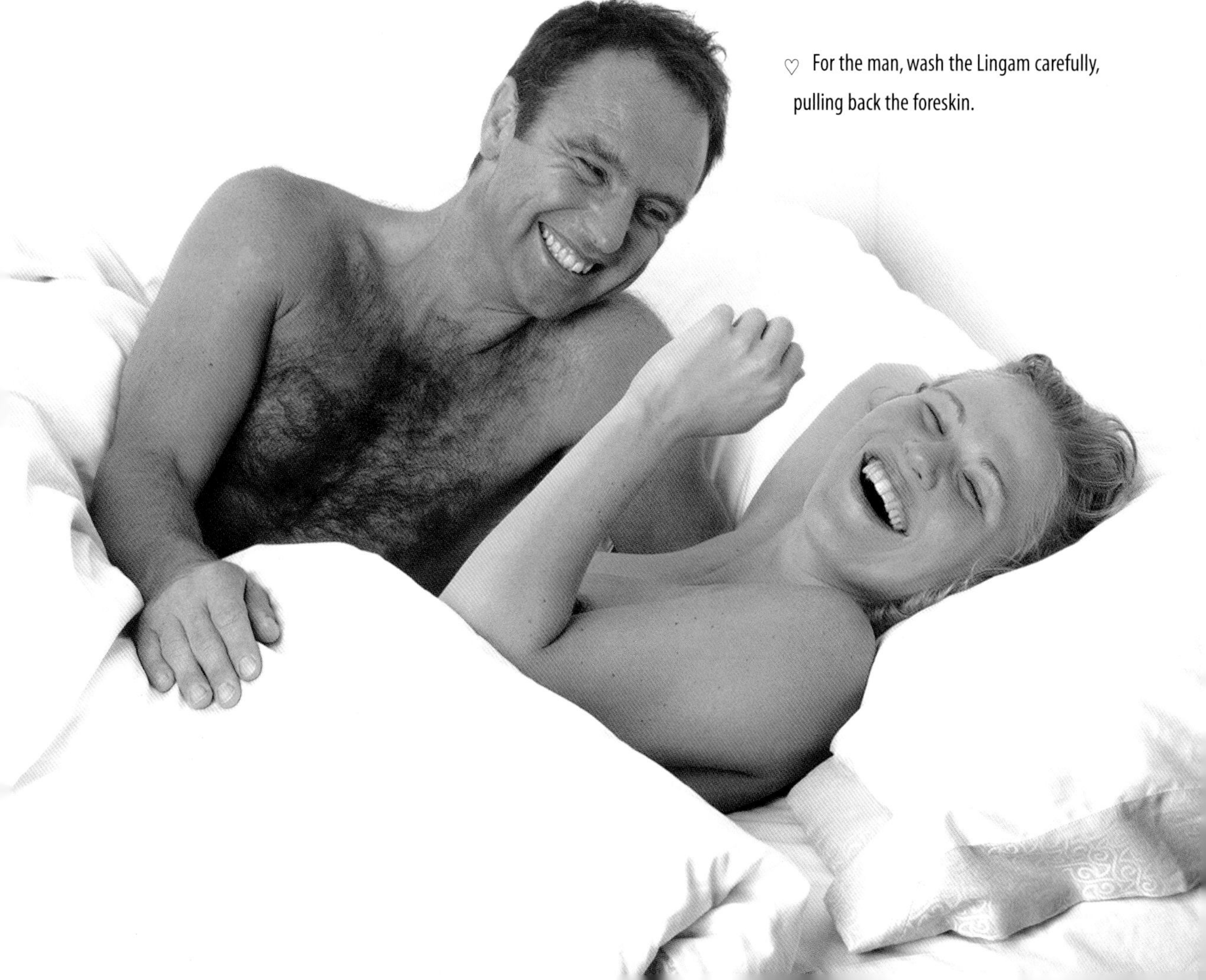

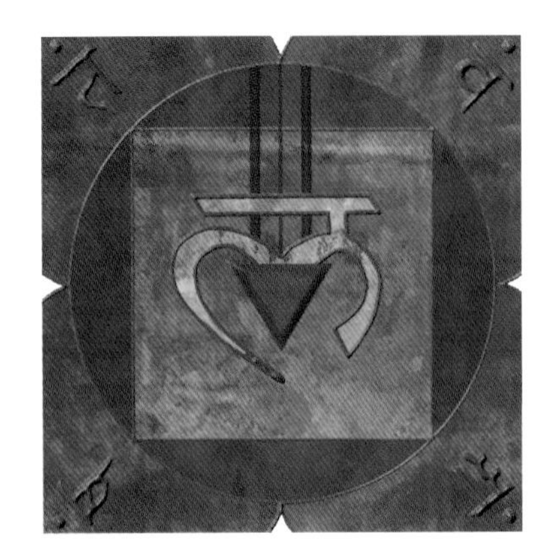

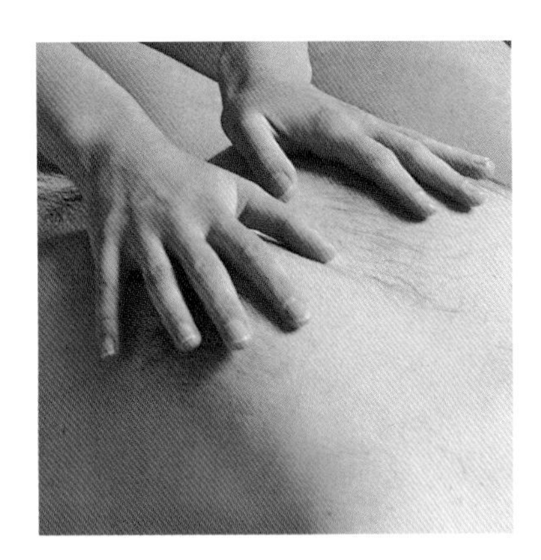

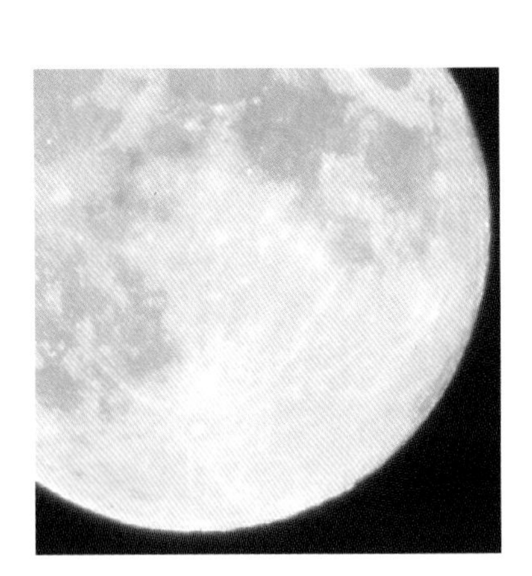

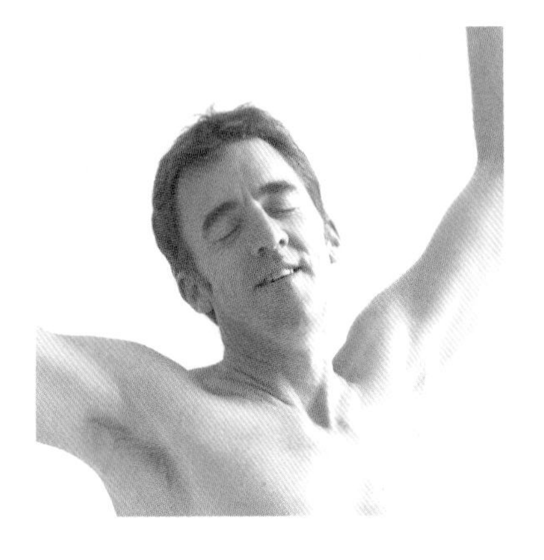

part 3
energy cycles

Subtle energy, a distillation of cosmic forces, is a mysterious guiding power in many facets of our lives. Exploring the impact of subtle energy in the chakra system, and how this affects male–female dynamics, leads you toward attaining oneness with a partner, sexually and spiritually. The "instructions" for becoming soul mates with a lover are encoded in the chakra system. Thus opening these with conscious touch and massage further expands your repertoire for becoming a master lover.

The moon has a tremendous impact on our bodies, emotions, and sexual cycles. Our body clocks are set to cosmic rhythms. By learning to tune into and absorb the wisdom in your hormonal cycle, you can honor and bring awareness to these cycles, and the more flowing and in tune with others and the rest of nature your life will become.

We are spirit made visible, and it is the challenge to honor this that gives depth and meaning to sexuality.

chapter 8

the chakra system

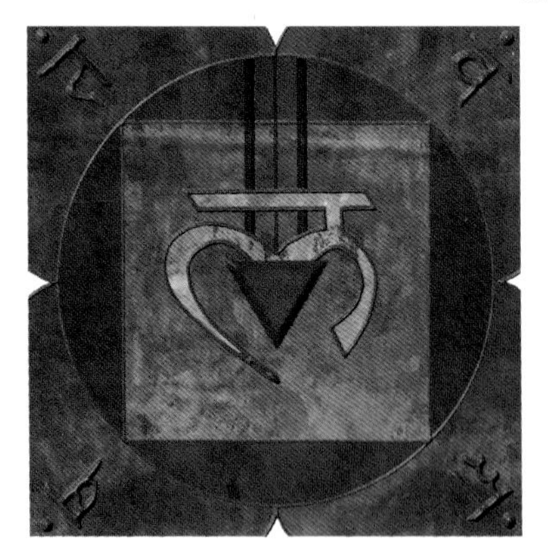

"As the man and the woman in me
Unite in love
The brilliance of beauty
Balanced on the bi-petaled lotus
Blooms in me"
Song from the Baul Mystics of Bengal, India,
translated by D Battacharya

Tantra supports the opening of the chakras into a flowing vertical system, uniting heaven and earth inside your being. If a man and woman can experience union together in all their six opposite and yet complementary centres (see pages 78–9), and are open to the vertical energy flow, their merging will be an experience of body, emotions, mind, soul, and spirit as one dynamic whole. As they are vibrating at one with the whole of themselves, it becomes natural and easy to vibrate in oneness together. This type of union is one of soul mates. It is an experience that can happen to any couple willing to join love and meditation in the practice of Tantra. What happens in sex is thus magnified to include the entire being, making the sex act a truly sensorial and spiritual awakening on all levels.

Chakra is a Sanskrit word meaning wheel. According to Eastern Mystical tradition, every person has seven chakras – centers of energy spinning like wheels, enabling pure life force to be absorbed. The chakras are along the central channel that runs vertically up the body from the coccyx to the top of the head.

These seven chakras hold the secret of how to attain awakened consciousness or spiritual liberation. The seeker of truth aspires to move on an inner journey through his or her chakra system, clearing energy stagnation and opening each center to its refined potential. Once this has been achieved in all seven chakras, the seven different frequencies of energy from the chakras merge, in the same way that the seven colors of light from the spectrum merge to create white light. This merging of the chakra energies leads to a state of consciousness called "enlightenment", or Mahamudra. The human being no longer relates to the world through a fragmented energetic system, but experiences the world through a sense of being one with all that is.

The energy of the chakras

In quantum physics theory, there is a dimension of energy that travels faster than the speed of light and has no frequency. Formless, yet holding the potential for all form, it is known as "zero point energy". From that dimension there is a step-down process into our world of matter and form. Pure life force energy (or Tachyon), which is linked to zero point energy, interfaces with matter by suffusing the subtle organizing energy field, or orbit, that exists around each particle of matter. A particle of matter infused with life force energy is able to expand into its potential of form. Thus cosmic energy continuously forms and interacts with the whole of the material world. Another way of viewing this is to think of zero point energy as spirit, life force energy (Tachyon) as the messenger of spirit, and the subtle organizing energy field around each life form as the soul.

Each chakra has a particular energy frequency and relates to the organs in the body that resonate with that frequency (seee pages 78–9). These organs absorb and distil this energy, and then radiate it out as a particular quality. Depending on the consciousness of the individual, what is radiated out is either in tune with that person's highest potential, or with energies that have yet to be purified in the alchemy of life. If an organ is vibrating in its refined potential, that chakra will be harmonious. Stagnation in a chakra is always associated with incomplete life experiences. Expression gets stuck in one way or another, and this leads to a blockage in the energy flow. There are many ways to open a flow in the chakra system, such as breath sessions, chakra massage, crystal healing, using Tachyonized products (see Resources, page 188), Tantra meditation, and in sessions using imagery and dialoguing.

"The invitation to make love through the energies of the different chakras was a gift in itself. To give over 'our' lovemaking to the very particular power of each center, and to let go of any idea or desires about what we might want or expect it to be like, was to experience vastly differing expressions of love and connection. It seemed as if each spoke louder to one or other of us, one becoming instinctively more 'active' and the other more receptive. It was only later that we realized that those corresponded with the positive poles within each of us."

Tim and Lindy, Tantra group participants

Positive and receptive poles

Each of the first six chakras have either Yin or Yang energy – they are either receptive (Yin) or positive (Yang) poles. The male and female chakra systems have opposite polarity except at the seventh chakra, which is beyond duality. The male and female chakra systems are described on pages 78–9. The Yin or receptive chakras can be compared to the negative pole of a magnet, while the Yang or emissive chakras can be compared to the positive pole. Between a man and a woman, the opposite polarities at each chakra attract each other, except at the seventh chakra where positive and receptive qualities are one. This simple understanding can revolutionize male–female relating.

Imbalances in these poles can lead to problems in relating, whether sexually or on day-to-day issues. It is important to remember that the Yin chakras open automatically if the Yang chakras are first awakened and opened. Positive pole massage, to awaken the Yang polarities, is described in chapter 9.

chakra energies

First chakra (sex center or root chakra)

In tune with the kidney, bladder, genitals, anus, pituitary gland, and male prostate. When the energy in this chakra is flowing freely, there is tremendous pleasure in sex.

Second chakra (navel center)

In tune with the liver, gallbladder, hypothalamus, and female uterus and ovaries. The navel is where you receive life from your mother in the womb. After birth, it is still an energetic link to the universal womb, the goddess. When the energy in this chakra flows freely there is joy and laughter; stagnation of energy here creates depression.

If this chakra is open and flowing during sex, the couple have a feeling of connection and a more profound experience of orgasm.

Third chakra (solar plexus)

In tune with the stomach, spleen, pancreas, lung, large intestine, the medulla oblongata, and the limbic system. This chakra digests new information and transforms it – here life experience becomes wisdom. In sex, when the couple's third chakras are open and flowing, they experience egolessness, and orgasm engulfs the whole body.

Fourth chakra (heart center)

Linked with the heart, small intestine, and thymus. The heart chakra purifies incomplete life experiences, seeking to distil everything in the crucible of love. It is here that conflict between lovers starts to evaporate. When lovers experience sexual union in this chakra, a quality of the sacred envelops them. Orgasm of the heart is divinely physical and yet carries a timeless mystical quality.

Fifth chakra (throat center)

In tune with the thyroid gland. This chakra is linked to the father, or male principle and is about the creative expression of truth and wisdom. Any unresolved issues around the male principle may cause energy stagnation in this chakra, leading to frustration. During orgasmic fusion between lovers in this chakra, the small self is burned in the fire of truth. The quality of orgasm is oceanic.

Sixth chakra (third eye)

Linked to the pineal gland, eyes, nose, and ears. If there is stagnation here, you live in a kind of spiritual sleep, not aware of the tremendous potential of life. Lovers uniting in this chakra may sense themselves as god and goddess. Their lovemaking becomes aware and sensitive, beyond time and mind. Orgasm here is an experience of unity, body and soul.

Seventh chakra (crown center)

Linked with the thalamus and the corpus callosum in the brain. The energy from this chakra radiates down through the whole body, through the central channel. Here is the union of inner male and female aspects, in perfect balance and attunement. When this chakra is open to the flow of universal energy during sex, the lovers are one undivided whole, merged with universal consciousness.

male polarities

The first chakra is a positive pole, shown physically by the way it "sticks out" from the body. A man's energy is naturally centered here and this chakra ignites energy for intercourse. This is where a man needs to feel loved. A loving touch will awaken the god residing in the Lingam and open the man's heart.

The second chakra is a more Yin, or receptive polarity of energy.

The third chakra is a positive pole. It is the seat of the soul. When a man radiates the power and strength of love from his solar plexus, the woman can receive it in her own third chakra, fulfilling a deep longing within her to be overtaken by male strength.

The fourth chakra is a receptive, Yin polarity.

The fifth chakra is a positive pole. From here the true male principle emanates, the creative expression of truth that arises from equilibrium of the first four chakras. As the woman's fifth chakra receives this energy, her love lifts to spiritual heights.

The sixth chakra is a receptive, Yin polarity.

The seventh chakra is beyond polarity. It is both Yin and Yang, and open to the supreme unity of male and female qualities.

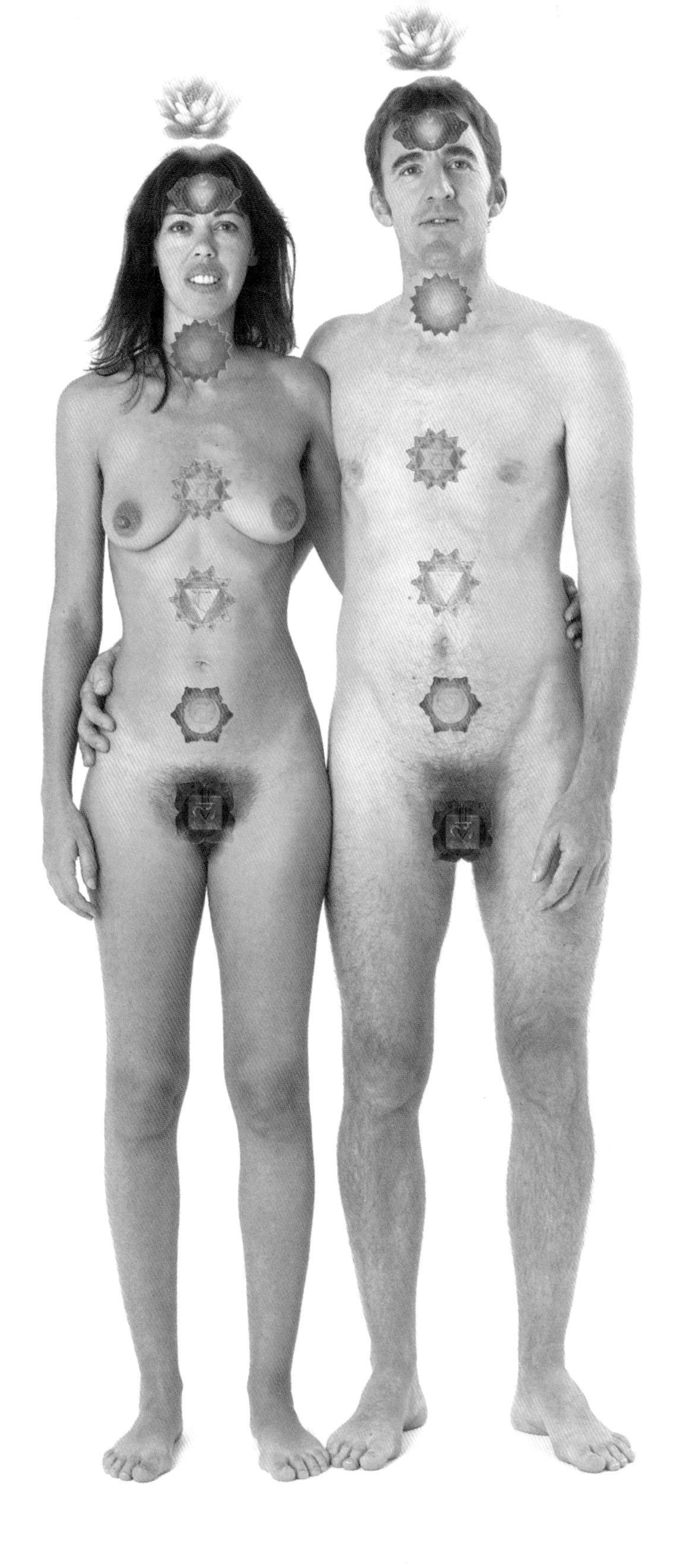

female polarities

The first chakra is a receptive, feminine, Yin polarity. This is shown physically by the way the woman's genitalia are mainly inside her body, and receptive to the male, Yang outward-going organ.

The second chakra is a positive pole. It is here that a woman's sexual energy naturally vibrates, and where she will create a child. When this chakra is open and flowing, it helps the man's second chakra to be receptive to her female sexuality, so that sex has a more profound sense of intimacy. It will also help her Yoni to become receptive to penetration and bring her a much richer orgasmic experience. This chakra is linked very powerfully to emotions, so the woman may laugh or cry as this chakra awakens.

The third chakra is a receptive, Yin polarity.

The fourth chakra is a positive pole. A woman is most centered on this chakra. It is here that the goddess resides and where she feels truly a woman. Massaging her breasts with loving and worshipping hands will awaken the goddess. Her love that emanates from this chakra will be so intoxicating that the man will fall in tune with it and relax into divine peace.

The fifth chakra is a receptive, Yin polarity.

The sixth chakra is a positive pole. Here the woman is in tune with the mysteries of existence. In Tantra the woman is considered as the initiator, because she channels and transmits this spiritual awakening to the man. Together they may then expand into the seventh chakra. Both souls melt as one, the highest potential of sex.

The seventh chakra is beyond polarity. It is both Yin and Yang, and open to the supreme unity of male and female qualities.

chakra dance meditation

This one-hour dance celebrates your life energy while opening your chakras. It is an active meditation, where bringing awareness to your body movements helps to create transformation.

♡ **Phase One:** Dance the quality of each chakra in turn, allowing seven minutes for each chakra (see the table of chakra qualities, right).

Begin at the first chakra, focusing on this chakra inside your pelvic region, radiating energy in all directions. Let your whole pelvis fill up with that energy, and dance from there. Then let your whole body be overtaken by the quality of the first chakra.

After seven minutes move your focus to the second chakra and again let the energy expand, as you dance the quality of that chakra, discovering what it is for you personally. Then allow that energy to engulf your whole body and become it, from head to toe, as you continue dancing.

Repeat for each chakra in turn, ending with the crown chakra.

♡ **Phase Two:** Lie down for 15 minutes, with eyes closed, simply witnessing your breathing, your mind, and your emotions as a detached observer. You may become aware of all seven chakras vibrating simultaneously.

We have produced a CD of music especially for this meditation (see Resources, page 188). Alternatively you can make your own, using seven minutes of music for each chakra. Make sure that the music you choose matches the quality of the given chakra.

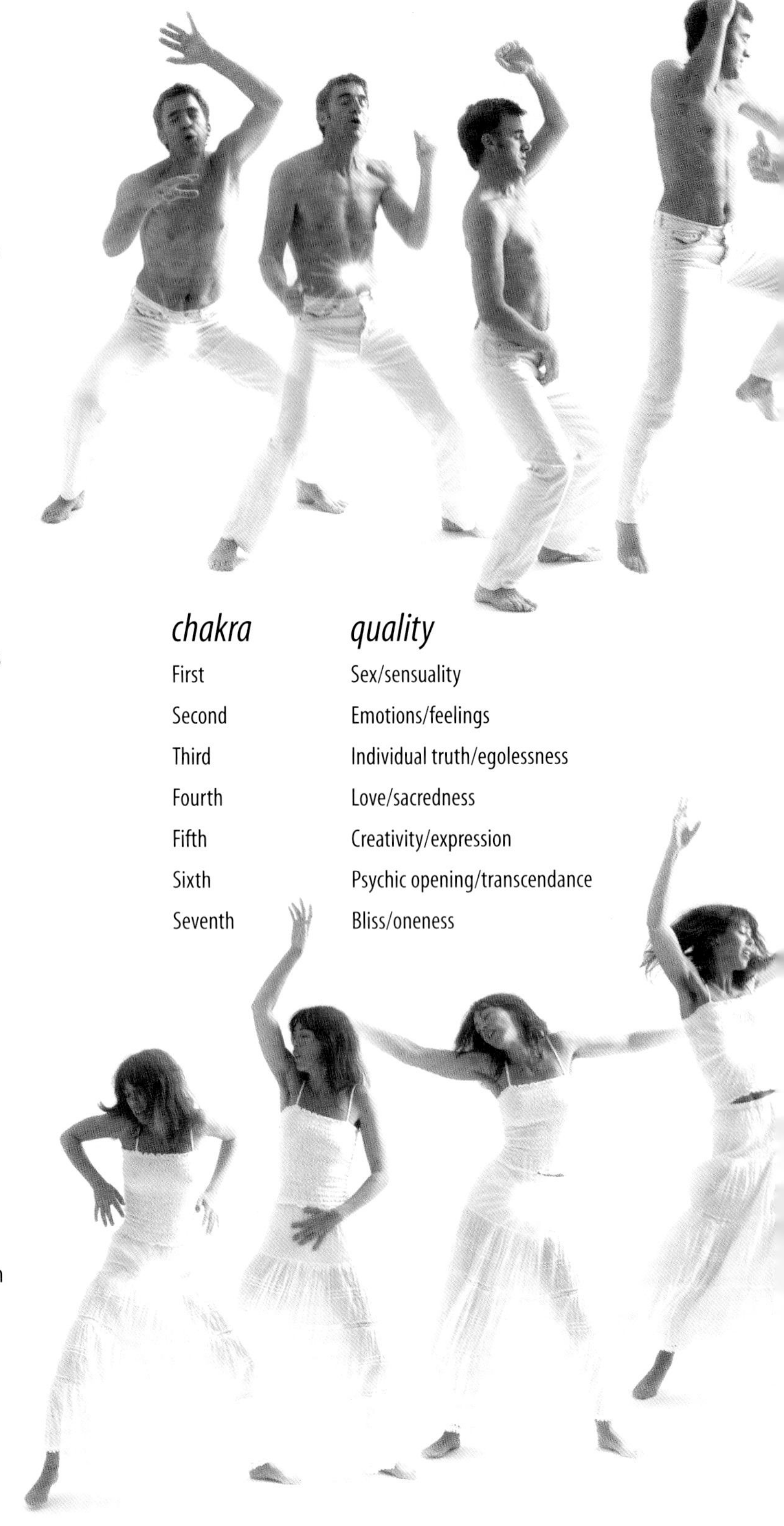

chakra	*quality*
First	Sex/sensuality
Second	Emotions/feelings
Third	Individual truth/egolessness
Fourth	Love/sacredness
Fifth	Creativity/expression
Sixth	Psychic opening/transcendance
Seventh	Bliss/oneness

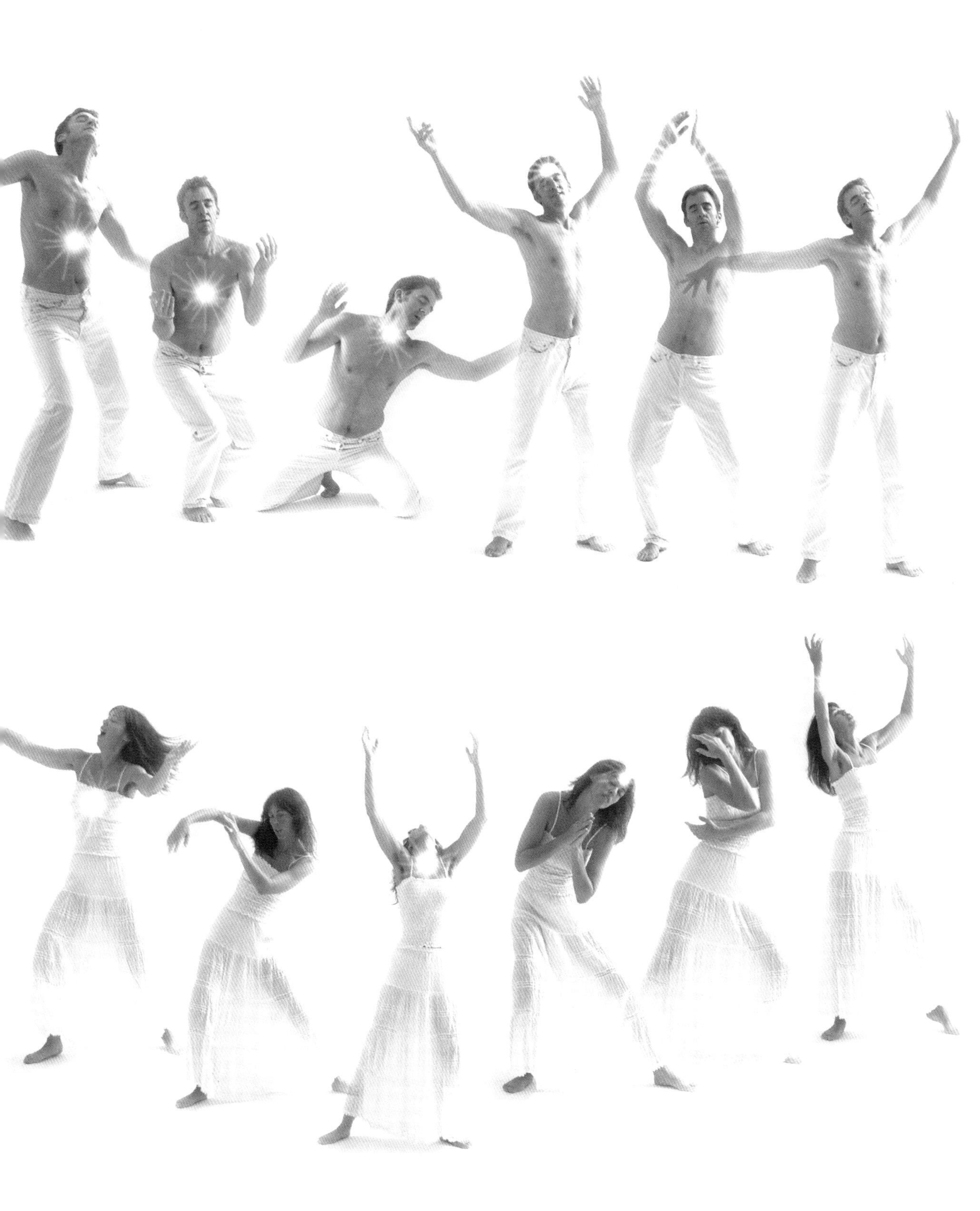

chapter 9

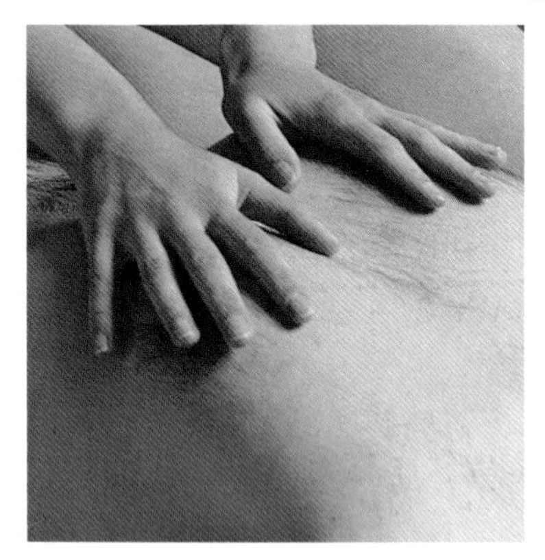

the language of touch

"Always remember God has no lips of his own, he kisses you through somebody else's lips. He has no hands of his own, he embraces you through somebody else's hands. He has no eyes of his own, because all eyes are his."
From *I Say Unto You Vol. 1*, Osho

Touch is almost a forgotten language in the larger part of our contemporary world. In many people's minds it has become synonymous with sex. This is a sign of a sexually "uneasy" and "out of touch" society.

Many people almost never receive or give a really nourishing touch. The body is viewed as a mechanism, with ideas of how it should look imposed upon it, according to the conditioning or fashion of the moment. More and more energy is directed to the mind, as if the mind were the only evolutionary human aspect. Everyday activities are carried out in a mechanical way, with no real physical awareness. Only when there is pain or disease do we become aware of our life in the body.

People have lost touch with the wisdom of the body. This wisdom is accessed through love and reverence for the miracle of life in this physical form. Pleasure, ecstasy, bliss, orgasm, natural instinctual intelligence, the thinking process (mind), intuition, inner knowing (gut feeling), wisdom, feelings (physical or emotional), and love are but a few of the qualities that can manifest only through our bodies. They bring an essential contribution to the meaning of life.

One of the special qualities of touch is its capacity to bring awareness to the body. For example, think of your sacrum, which you may not be aware of in this moment. The simple touch of a hand there will bring your awareness to this area and allow you to experience this body part and the subtle sensations or qualities associated with it. As we tend to go up in our heads and disconnect with the body, touch is the most effective way of helping us to "come down" into the body. The development of awareness and sensitivity of the body is a prerequisite for the expansion of love and ecstasy in our lives.

expressions of touch

♡ Touch that conveys love, tenderness, affection, and care is a Yin type of touch, drawing on female qualities (whether given by men or women). This type of touch is the most forgotten nowadays. The hands are relaxed as they touch or caress the beloved. As most of us do not receive enough touch in childhood, we are not fluid, or we feel awkward with this method of expression. Days or weeks go by without it, until we reach a point of "touch starvation", though often we are not even aware of this lack.

♡ Sexual touch is used to turn on the partner before and during penetration. This type of touch is the most commonly given nowadays – people seldom touch for non-sexual reasons. This type of touch has a more Yang or male quality. It communicates desire.

♡ The healing touch reconnects you to the whole. Many healing traditions are based on an understanding that the physical body is a dynamic process in the energy continuum (see chapter 8), and discoveries in modern physics are confirming this. Healing takes place when a person is reconnected to and able to absorb source energy. The healer and his or her hands channel the healing force to the receiver.

♡ Conscious touch propels the giver and receiver into a circle of energy where both the partners disappear into an experience of the here and now: an open door into the great mysteries of life. The bodies lose their density and become more like fluid energies. The Lover and Beloved melt together as one undivided whole.

The hands

The hands are marvellously sensitive instruments of communication. A simple touch will convey much. That is because the hands are strongly connected to the brain – they are almost like branches of the mind. We observe this in the way that people's hand movements accompany their speech, gesticulating and illustrating what they say. Even when someone is thinking, their thoughts show their hand movements. When you touch another person, your hands will convey the thoughts or desires that are in your mind, and the receiver will somehow interpret these on a physical level and sense the intention behind the touch. This is what we mean by "the language of touch".

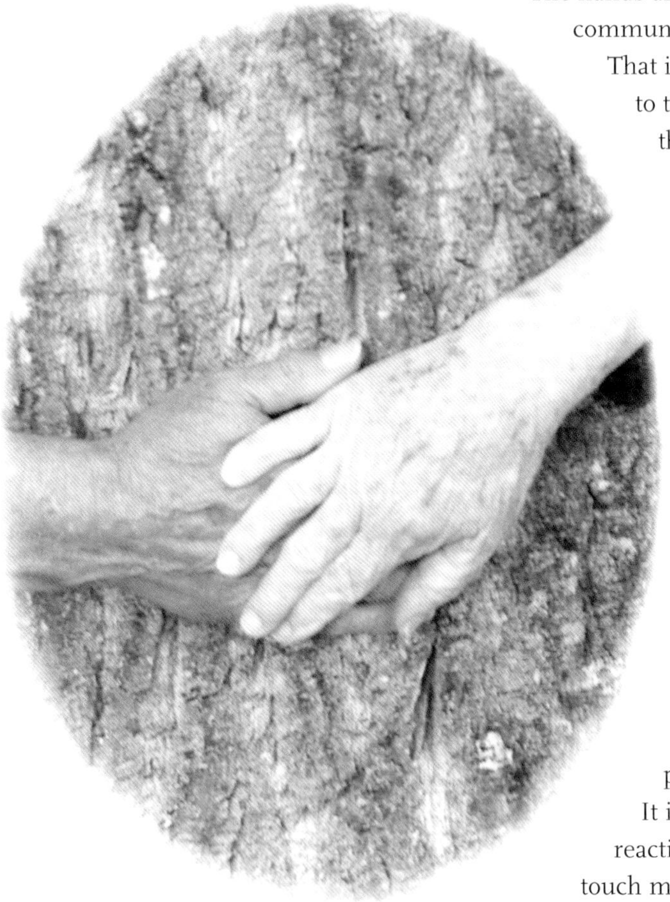

Between lovers, as the relationship settles, touch is mainly used to create excitement in lovemaking. This type of touch is right for the communication of passion, the desire for fusion and orgasm. It is a goal-oriented touch, given solely to get a reaction from the partner. Although this kind of touch may be appropriate for creating a moment of hot and passionate sex, it does not help to generate the expansion of feminine qualities. The feminine polarities in men and women are awakened in different ways (see chapter 8), but for both, it is helpful if touch is given with the hands and mind relaxed.

Massage and caress your partner with relaxed and loving hands that carry no agenda from the mind of an end goal or a desired outcome. Your touch will then be a sharing of overflowing love, tenderness, appreciation, and gratefulness. To get into that relaxed, tender, and loving mood, it is helpful to have the framework of a massage or Tantra method.

Massage with a lover

When exchanging a massage with your lover, technique is not so important. What makes all the difference is giving loving, conscious touch. Focus on the touch you give, be present in it and joyful. Being present means that the partner giving the massage is fully aware in the moment of what he or she is doing. Remember that whatever is in your mind will be transmitted through your hands to your partner. So observe your mind as you give the massage. When you become aware that it is engaged in thoughts or moods, just come back to feelings of love and gratefulness.

Most importantly, when you give the massage, enjoy it. If you are enjoying it, your partner will enjoy it too, because a circle of giving and receiving is created between you. Giving and receiving are two complementary opposites – you cannot have one without the other. If you feel depleted after giving, it means that you are not truly giving – you are holding back and so are unable to receive fully either. If you can come back again and again to your enjoyment in giving the massage, the circle between you of simultaneous giving and receiving will take you both into a space of deep and soul-nourishing intimacy.

When you consciously remain present in the moment, giving or receiving pleasurable touch, you enter into an experience of the eternal. This moment, lived with awareness, is beyond time and mind, and thus becomes a doorway into infinity. Such an experience is what many people are searching for when they enter into lovemaking. But since there is usually no teaching for how to bring it about, it only happens rarely. Cultivating the skills of conscious touch can bring you this life-enhancing and nurturing experience more often.

"Because I have been practicing and teaching massage for years, touch has been very much a part of my life. As I started to learn more about touch, I realized that it was an art that had nothing to do with massage techniques or other bodywork methods I had been trained in. It was more to do with how relaxed and present I was with myself. I found that my hands were incredible tools for meditation, because observing them would reveal my state of mind, and my desire to heal or please. All desires bring tension into the hands.

Touch is so simple, but the mind does not believe it can be so. Touch in itself is enough. It is miraculous in its simplicity and effect. It helps us connect in a profound and intimate way to others and ourselves."

Geho

positive poles massage

In this massage, you exchange a massage with your partner, using conscious touch that communicates love and gratefulness. During the massage you also focus on each of your partner's positive poles (see page 78–9) in turn and then integrate this energy through the whole body. This will help your partner's chakra system to come into its natural resonance, which will powerfully affect the magnetism between you.

Take turns to massage each other. Then you will be ready to enter into lovemaking from a place of heightened sensitivity, balance, and openness.

♡ Start on your partner's back, using the techniques described on page 36 to awaken the sacral area and then guiding that energy up, and opening the spine by stroking up either side of it. Then massage the back of the head lightly. Next massage the backs of the legs and the feet.

♡ Ask your partner to turn over and then start to massage the front of the legs and the feet. Next focus on the inner thighs all the way up to the groin. Then follow the instructions for either the man or the woman, as appropriate.

Massage for the man:

♡ Massage the belly softly, making clockwise movements around the navel. Then focus on the solar plexus (3rd chakra) between the rib cage and the navel. Complete the massage in this area by resting your relaxed hands for some moments on the solar plexus.

♡ Integrate the solar plexus energy into the rest of the body by stroking again around the whole belly and then stroking upward, letting your hands glide up and out along the shoulders, arms, and hands.

Massage the arms and hands, and then come back to the neck and throat (5th chakra). Finish by resting one hand on the neck while the other rests lightly on the throat.

♡ Massage the head, including the face, scalp, and ears.

♡ Massage around the genitals at the groin and around where they are attached to the body (1st chakra). Then focus on the perineum point between the testicles and the anus.

Next massage the Lingam and testicles and cradle them in your hands. As you touch the Lingam, remember that the name Lingam means "pillar of light". The emphasis is not on exciting your partner, but on loving, honoring, and relaxing tensions in that area. It does not matter whether or not your partner has an erection. Just enjoy the miracle of the male principle as embodied in this Lingam.

♡ To complete the massage, integrate the energy from the genitals with the rest of the body by stroking down the legs and up the body, through the chest, across the shoulders, and along the arms. Then rest your palms very lightly over the eyes for a few moments, allowing your partner to let go into a deeply nourishing silent space. Finally lift your hands up and away from his body; then you can Namaste to each other as a sign of gratitude (see page 100).

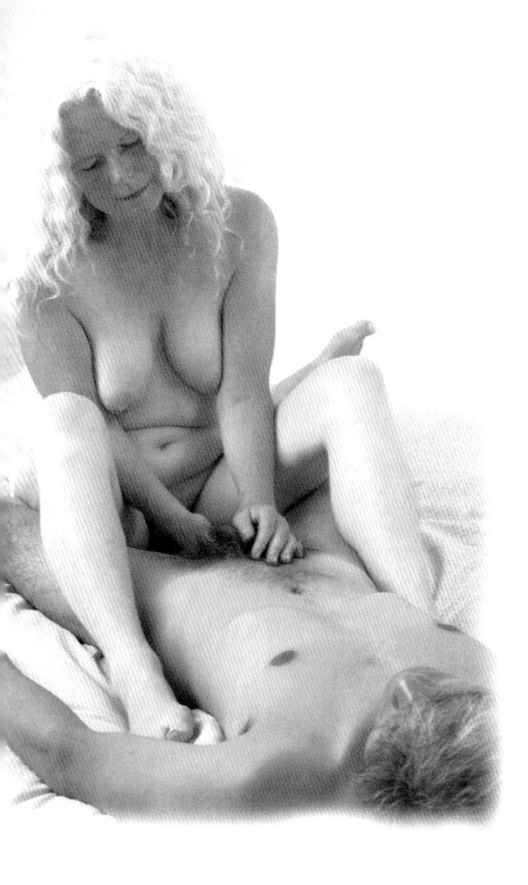

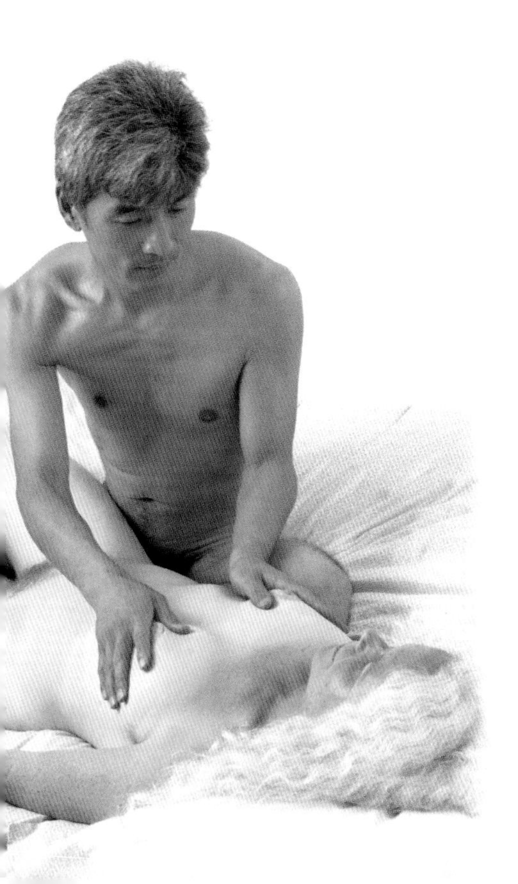

Massage for the woman:

♡ Massage the belly lightly and lovingly, with gentle movements clockwise around the navel. Then rest your relaxed hands here, covering the area between the pubic hair line and the navel (2nd chakra) for a couple of minutes.

♡ Integrate the belly's energy with the rest of the body by stroking upward over the chest (4th chakra) and out along the arms and hands. Massage the breasts. (It may be helpful to ask the woman to show you how she likes to have her breasts massaged, before you begin this massage.) As you massage her breasts, the emphasis is not on turning her on, but on honoring her as a goddess and drawing nourishment and love from them. Finish by stroking the awakened energy around the breasts out through the arms and hands.

♡ Massage the arms and hands and then move up to the neck, scalp, and face. Stroke all over the neck, scalp, and ears and then the face. Focus on the forehead and between the eyebrows (6th chakra). Caress upward from the bridge of the nose to the hairline softly and repeatedly for a couple of minutes, to open the third eye.

♡ Start massaging lightly around the Yoni and the groin area (1st chakra), then softly caress the Yoni and pubic hair, with great adoration and respect, remembering that Yoni means "sacred place". Use loving touch at the opening of the Yoni and on the clitoris. Your emphasis is not on arousing the woman, but on loving her.

♡ To complete the massage, integrate the energy from the genitals with the rest of the body by stroking down the legs and up the body, through the chest, across the shoulders, and along the arms. Then rest your relaxed hands on the belly, below the navel, for a few moments. When you feel her sinking deeper into let go, you can slowly lift your hands off the body and into the aura, allowing the 2nd chakra to expand even more. Lift your hands up and away from her body; then you can Namaste to each other as a sign of gratitude (see page 100).

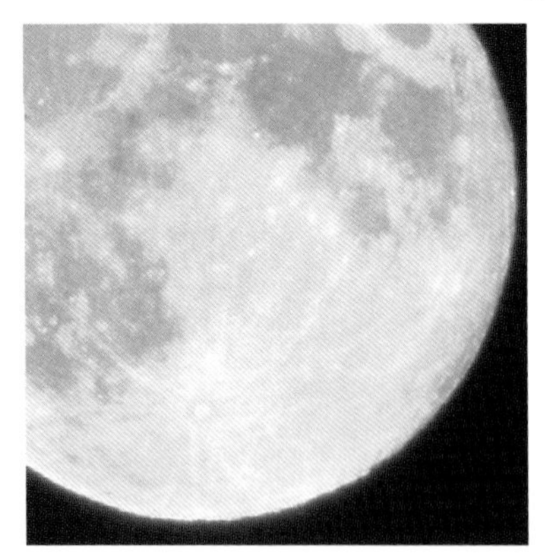

the female sexual cycle

"The sea was the Mother
The Mother was not people, she was not anything.
Nothing at all
She was when she was, darkly
She was memory and potential
She was Aluna"
From the oral creation story of the Kogi Indians of Columbia, translated by Alan Ereira

If women could learn to tune into and live according to their nature, what a relaxed, joyous, and loving world this would be. For the woman is the custodian of time, the seasons, and the rhythm of life. Her body is the clock that sets the whole world in motion; with her rest the secrets of birth, life, love, and death. This is why ancient societies respected and revered the feminine.

According to ancient Tantra texts, a woman's natural rhythm is to ovulate with the full moon and menstruate with the new moon. Also, each phase of the moon is linked with one aspect of the goddess, incorporating 16 goddess aspects in all. A man studying the way of Tantra would meditate on the woman's Yoni, observing the effect of the goddess cycles in her energy, and thus learning to fall in tune with the whole of creation.

In our society, women are in the process of regaining the feminine power inherent in the moon's cycle. According to ancient Indian scriptures, humanity is currently at the end of a long cycle of ignorance known as the Kali Yuga, which will be followed by a new age of wisdom and enlightenment (see chapter 27). Because we are still cocooned in the Kali Yuga, we stumble over the programming of previous generations. One example of this is that many women are not in touch with their moon cycles, and do not know when they are ovulating, when their sexual desire is at its peak, or when they simply need nurturing. Many women have sex only to receive a little tender touch. They may go for orgasm aggressively when their bodies are not asking for it, just to experience some relief from tension.

Women's bodies have become confused, due to unhealthy eating habits, or through medication that upsets hormonal balance, such as the birth control pill. This prevents the woman experiencing the wonder of her body as it progresses through her natural monthly cycle, because it alters that cycle into a synthetic replica of the real thing.

An unhealthy lifestyle also has a disastrous effect on the menopause, which nowadays is treated as if it is a disease.

five phases of the monthly cycle

The woman, like the sea, is receptive to the waxing and waning of the moon. Her monthly cycle is divided into five phases.

From the end of menstruation to the 10th day of the cycle (counting day 1 as the first day of menstruation), the woman is hormonally and psychologically like a young girl. She may want to play and flirt, without needing to consummate the love act with penetration. She will enjoy being stroked, caressed, and kissed.

From the 10th to the 18th day she is in the phase of young womanhood. This is her fertile phase, when she is most likely to conceive. During this time, one of her ovaries releases an egg that travels to the fallopian tube to await possible fertilization. At this time the woman is ready for passionate lovemaking with many orgasms, and to explore different sexual positions. At ovulation she releases a clear, slippery, and juicy mucus in her vagina, which helps the sperm to swim toward the egg. It also acts as a lubricant during sex, and has an aphrodisiac odor to arouse the man.

From the 18th day until four days before menstruation the woman is in the phase of middle age, which is a phase of meditation, self-contemplation, and liberation. Lovemaking using Tantra methods for enhancing intimacy and for spiritual uplifting will nourish her.

From four days before the beginning of menstruation until menstruation begins is the pre-menstrual flush. This is similar to the time before death, when all the energies of life come together for a final burst of creativity. This creativity carries in it all that the woman has lived in the past month. If she has not lived her potential she may feel miserable, physically and psychologically. If she has lived her energy freely, a sudden rush of life force will propel her into expression of some kind – spring-cleaning the house, jumping on her man for passionate sex, or undertaking artistic projects.

When menstruation begins, there is a sudden drop in hormone levels, and a loss of energy. The lining of the womb, which was designed to be the nest for a possible new life, is released and flows out through the Yoni. This is the phase of de-creation, death, let go. In this phase the woman needs to rest and meditate, relaxing deeply into the valley, there to be washed clean of all impurities that may have gathered during the previous month. The first two days of menstruation are often accompanied by an aching in the lower back, cramping in the womb, and aching in the legs. These are clear signals from the body that it is time to rest. After that, as menstruation continues, full-body massage will help to release toxins and soothe aches and pains.

The main flow of blood lasts for around three days and then tapers off for two more days, although for some women it lasts longer. If you use pads to catch the blood rather than tampons, you have the opportunity to feel more in tune with the phases of your flow. In Aboriginal societies and in ancient matriarchal cultures it was normal practice for women having their menstrual period to get together to rest and relax. They were not expected to work at that time. In our society women need to create a lifestyle in which this time of the month can be honored.

If a woman feels like making love and sharing this precious time with her lover then she should use the female on top position, to allow the full flow of her blood to descend on to the man. The man is then receptive to the powerful teaching about death and renewal that the woman's body and psyche emit at this time. The Baul mystics, a society of wandering Tantric adepts in India, hold monthly ritual celebrations at the time of the new moon for men to become empowered by the woman's menstrual flow. It is their understanding that during the last 12 hours of the menstrual flow they will receive the most beneficial transmission from a woman during sexual union.

Instead of looking forward to this time of liberation and wisdom, women dread it as a painful and debilitating passage into defeat and old age. In societies where women eat a balanced diet and older women are respected, menopause is an easy and natural transition into the full moon of life. Freed of the responsibilities she may have had when younger, the woman has the opportunity to become playful and serene at the same time.

Living by the moon's rhythms

A woman's nature is receptive. She is a conduit, a passage, for a soul to be born. She has the quality of a medium, open and receptive to what will manifest through her; whatever manifests in our human world is born through women. If a woman is unconscious she can be used as a medium for the ills of the world, through her passive co-operation. If she is in tune with the universal laws and awakens to love, she will become the conduit for the healing and the renewal of the planet. No man can start a war or create any kind of mischief in the world without the passive co-operation of women.

The more women regain their moon cycle with its inherent obedience to universal laws, the sooner our human societies will come into balance. One way to do this would be to revert to the moon calendar, first used by the Mayans. This single change would empower the feminine and thus transform society.

When women gather together, feminine moon energy is enhanced. At women-only gatherings you can celebrate the feminine in belly dancing, massage, bathing, and sharing about subjects close to your heart. You could set up study groups to learn more about feminine sexuality, conception, birth, child-raising, health, the environment, Tantra, and the awakening of the goddess. The more women participate in these gatherings, the more there will be an energetic balance between Yin and Yang in the world.

becoming a moon goddess

♡ Purchase a moon calendar and display it in a prominent place.

♡ Keep a moon diary. Note your moods, and keep a record of your physical changes throughout the month, for example, at ovulation, and before and during menstruation. Record the fluctuations in your sexual energy. At what times do you desire orgasm? When do you yearn for cuddling rather than sex? When are you flirty?

♡ Compare your findings with the cycles of the moon. In this way you may slowly gain insight into your moon rhythms and what they mean for you. The more you respect these natural rhythms, the more relaxed and happy you will be.

♡ Whenever you have a chance, find a place in nature where you can be in the night and tune into the moon. Dance naked under the full moon or have a moon bath, just resting and receiving moon energy.

♡ Invite other women to keep a moon diary, and get together to share your findings.

♡ Have moonlight goddess celebrations.

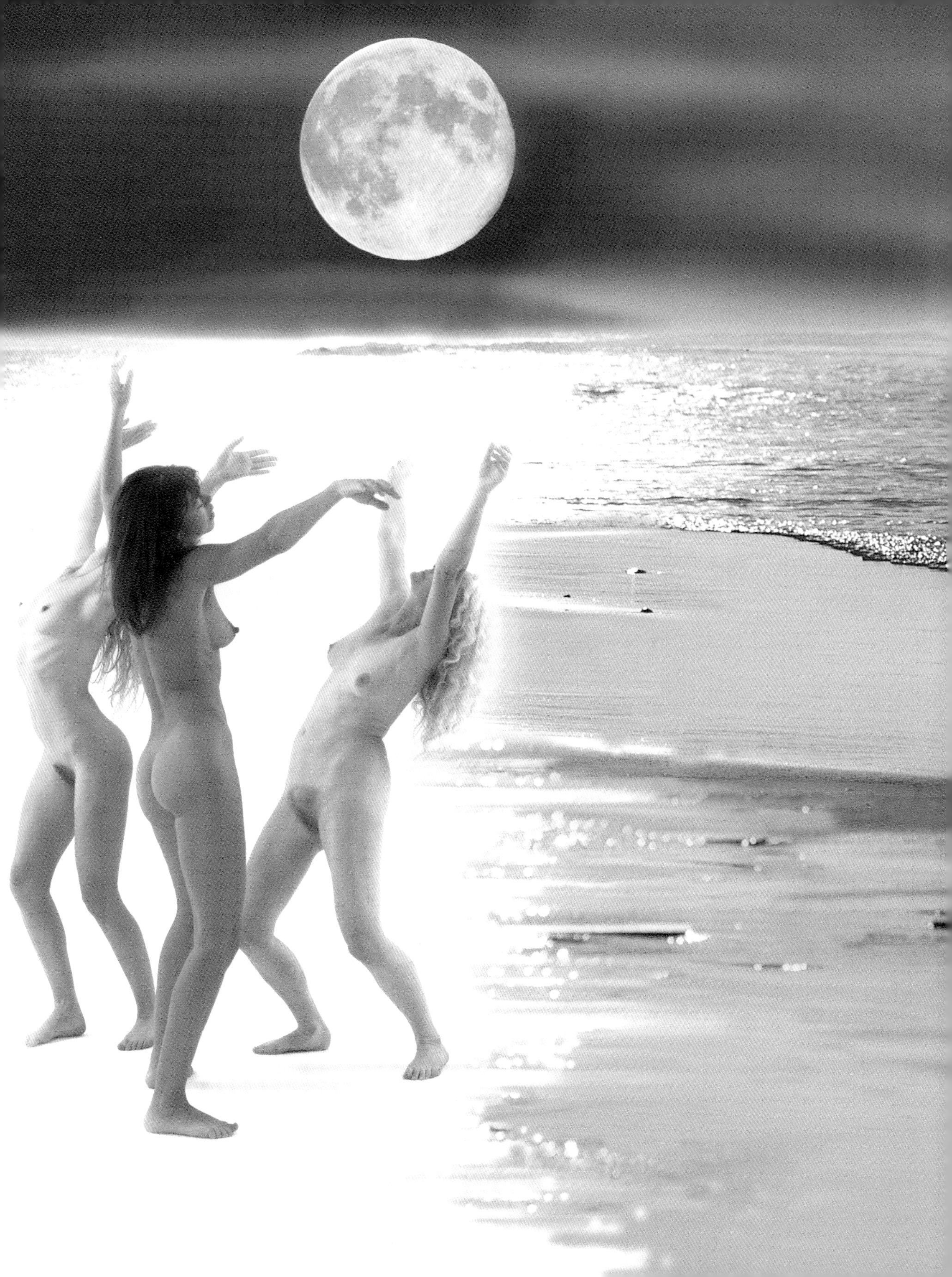

chapter 11

the male sexual cycle

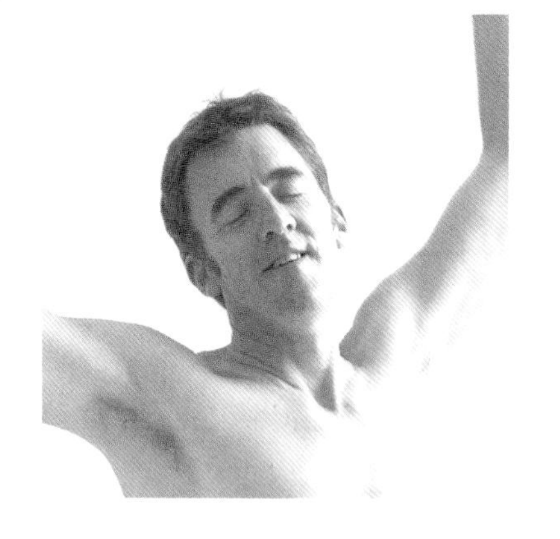

"The man is not less the soul, nor more
He too is in his place, he too is all qualities
He is action and power ...
... The wildest largest passions
... He brings everything to the test of himself
... He strikes soundings at last only here"
From *I Sing the Body Electric* (1867) Walt Whitman

If men can hold this one golden key, it will open the doors of paradise here on earth. Let all your power, strength, intellect, and creativity be focused on a single goal: how to nurture, protect, and serve the feminine life qualities of love, compassion, devotion to life, appreciation of art, aesthetics, beauty, health consciousness, and refined sensitivity.

Male and female both instinctively seek wholeness, where the male and female polarities are in complementary unity. This instinct is the biological remembrance of the shared origin of male and female life.

The female egg carries an X chromosome. Some male sperm carry an X chromosome, others carry a Y chromosome. When a sperm carrying the X chromosome penetrates the egg, the resulting child develops into a girl (XX); if the sperm carries the Y chromosome the child will be a boy (XY). At the beginning there is no difference between male and female foetuses. Then at six or seven weeks' gestation, the testis determining factor on the male Y chromosome becomes active, and the foetus begins to develop male genitalia. Thus the feminine, or X blueprint, is the foundation for human life. The male, Y blueprint arises as a complementary polarity to the feminine. So in a deep sense the male sex cycles are in response to the feminine, bonded to her like lock and key.

Hormonal cycles

A man's primary developmental and sexual impulses are fuelled by testosterone. This hormone gives rise to the male qualities of action, adventurousness, aggressiveness, creative impulses, competitiveness, protectiveness, a need for hierarchy, clear structures, and boundaries, and abundant libido. It is also responsible for male body characteristics: large frame, muscular strength, height, hairiness, and a deep voice.

At puberty testosterone levels rise by about 800 per cent, creating dramatic physical, emotional, and sexual changes. The

a man's moon cycle

A man's monthly cycle is less clearly defined than a woman's and does not interfere with his ability to release sperm. Nature has made sure that he is ever ready to impregnate a woman. However, men do report a regular cycle, incorporating a monthly drop in energy levels, a phase of emotional turmoil, and times in the month where they feel more highly sexed. It would be surprising if it were not so, since each man carries a shadow side of himself that is feminine, just as every woman carries a shadow side that is masculine.

The male monthly cycle takes its cues from the moon. The phase of no moon leading into new moon is analogous to a woman's menstruation, a two-day period when the man may need to be alone and introspective. He may have lower energy levels and feel the need to pamper himself in some way. During the next phase, lasting about four days, he may feel soft, tender, and romantic. This then leads into an 11-day phase of build-up of sexual energy, peaking around the time of the full moon and analogous to a woman's ovulation. At this time his creative genius can flower. In the final phase, from the full moon until about two days before the new moon, the man may feel more settled within himself, able to relate to others from a place of balance, and less driven by the demands of his reproductive urges. These phases can be seen as phases of the child, the adolescent, the adult, and the older man, or as innocence, creativity, fulfilment, and introspection, leading to wisdom, death, and rebirth.

keeping a monthly journal

It may bring you great insight to keep a monthly diary, recording how you feel at each change of the moon in your sexuality, your physical health, your emotions and moods, and your thoughts and fantasies. However, your cycles may not necessarily relate to the changes in the moon as described left, since urban cultures are not usually attuned to the moon's cycles.

As more men and women experiment with keeping track of their cycles, relations between male and female will become more harmonious. If you read chapter 10 on female sexual cycles, you will see that men and women are both programmed in a similar way, and have similar needs and urges according to changes in the moon. A better understanding of these cycles will amplify a balanced sexuality.

the sun cycle

The sun is in tune with the fiery qualities of testosterone and also influences men's bodies and behavior. Every 11 years there is an increase in the number of solar flares (eruptions of high-energy radiation from the sun's surface) and during this time war and violence among men are more likely. It has also been noted that at such times men's blood becomes thinner.

The sun also has a 90-year cycle, rising to a peak of activity through 45 years and then decreasing into a valley for the next 45 years. During the movement toward the peak, humans are more healthy. With the descent into the valley, there is more likelihood of outbreaks of disease, dramatic climatic changes, and earthquakes.

"The more I am fluid with my emotions, the more I truly feel my heart and see that love reflected back in others."

Michael, Tantra group participant

adolescent boy feels the urge to ejaculate frequently and may have erections at any time. Physically, a man reaches his sexual peak at the age of 18. If he can act on his impulse to have sex within wise boundaries, such as those of Tantra, he will discover the heights his hormones can bring him to and that sex opens the door to love and superconsciousness.

The Kogi Indians of Columbia, an ancient hidden civilization only recently discovered living in the Sierra Nevada, believe that women do not need to be taught spirituality because they are already the embodiment of the essence of life. The Kogi are very meticulous in the spiritual discipline given to men, as they believe that men, if not properly trained, can more easily lose their way and find themselves in a confused state of mind, torn between diverse aspects of themselves.

From the age of 19 to about 40, testosterone levels remain fairly constant. This gives the man the opportunity to become comfortable with and refine who he is, mentally, emotionally, and sexually. After 40, testosterone levels slowly decrease and he may feel less driven by ambition, more in tune with the feminine, and have more understanding of life in its wholeness.

As long as a man's creative power is in the service of the feminine qualities of love and compassion, he is using his attributes in accordance with the laws of nature. If he starts to dominate the feminine he cuts himself off from his own roots. For a boy's male qualities to find a positive direction as he grows up, he needs clearly defined boundaries, from an authority based on love and compassion.

Emotional states

A man is under constant pressure to prove himself sexually, to prove his abilities as a provider for his family, to prove himself as a wise father and loyal husband, to prove himself as a good tax-payer to his country, and sometimes to be ready to die for a cause he may not even understand. He may experience peace only within the arms of a caring woman, who loves and accepts him as he is. Men's emotion rarely finds an easy outlet, since many societies frown upon a man who is emotional. If a man's tears (whether of joy or sadness) are not allowed, this repressed energy may move toward anger, violence, or addictive behaviour.

Our society's repression of male emotions and ignorance of the male hormonal cycle are some of the reasons why war is so common. War is only possible when natural outlets of energy – naturally flowing sexuality and emotions – are blocked. All the exercises in this book help to free sexual and emotional flow. From a flowing, sensitive energy comes harmonious relating with other people and a feeling of being at home in oneself.

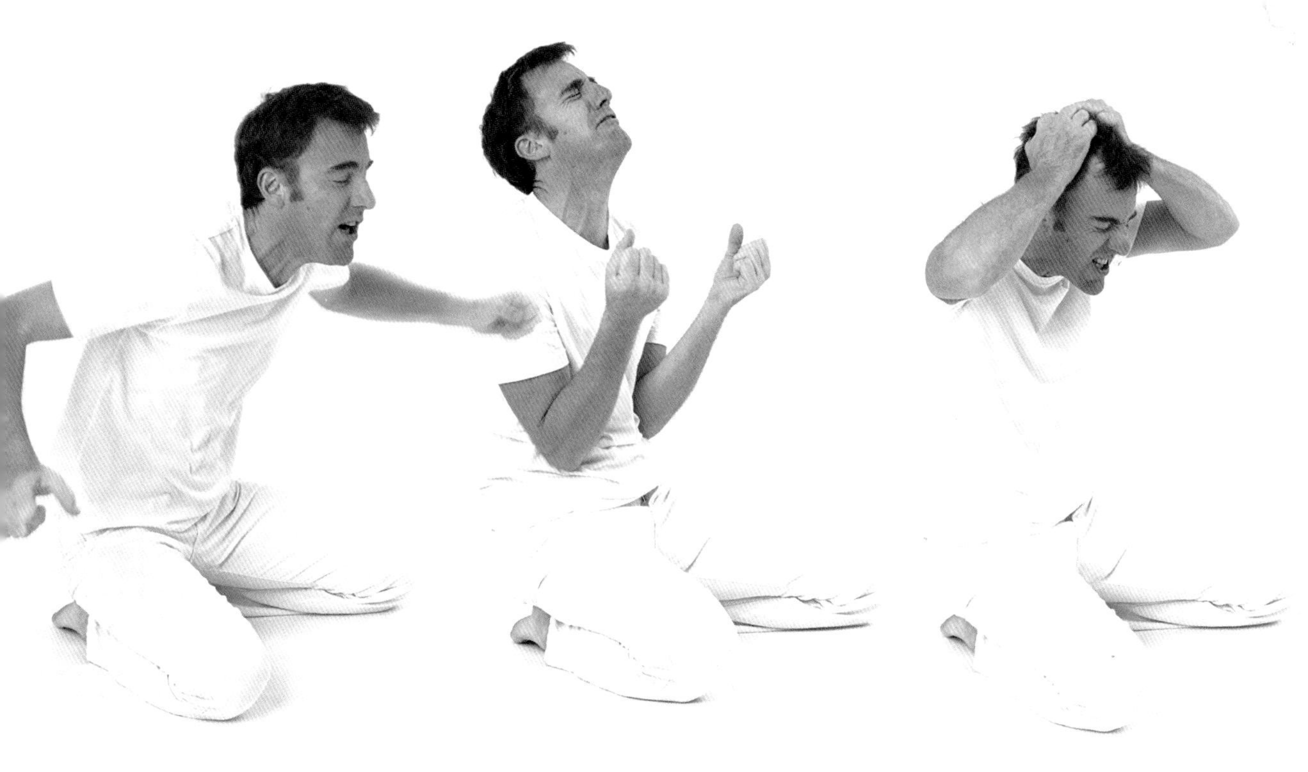

becoming the emotion

This simple exercise is truly liberating for both men and women. Do it alone, to allow yourself more freedom of expression. By stimulating emotional fluidity, the exercise will help you to become freer with who you really are, and to feel more balanced. Allowing yourself to become your emotions totally for a fixed amount of time allows you then to dive deeper into serenity.

♡ **Phase one:** (30 minutes) Become your present mood or your emotion. Pull all kinds of faces. Let your body take different postures, to portray how you feel.

For example, you can become rage itself, throttle a cushion, or jump up and down, roll your eyes, grimace, make sounds. Or you may become sadness, weep, curl up in a ball, be miserable. Become laughter, give a good belly laugh, roll on the floor, legs in the air as you laugh, and so on. You don't have to invent moods, just indulge, let go, amplify and act out what is there inside you moment by moment during the 30 minutes. During that time your moods and emotions may shift several times, or they may not.

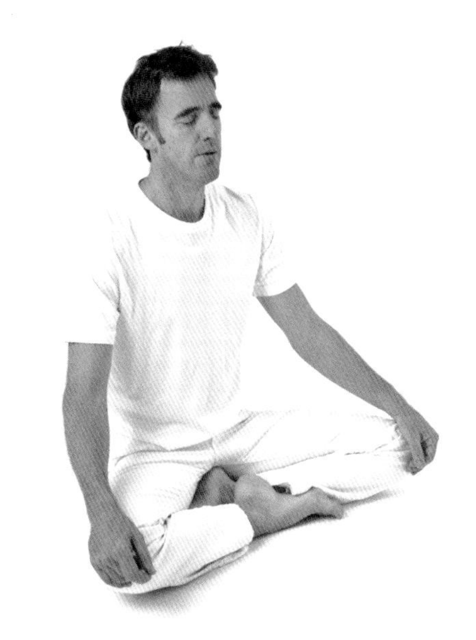

♡ **Phase two:** (30 minutes) Either sit with a straight back or lie down, eyes closed, in silence. Just become a witness of your body, your mind, and your emotions, a detached observer in the drama of life.

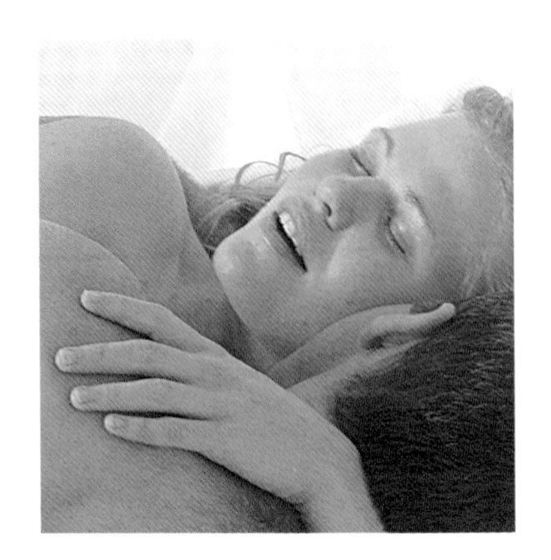

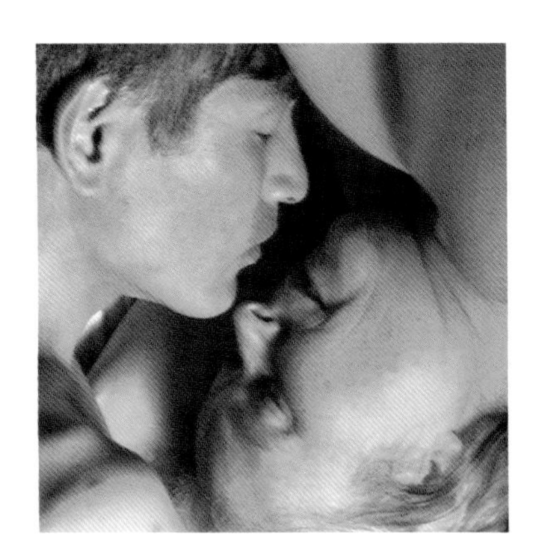

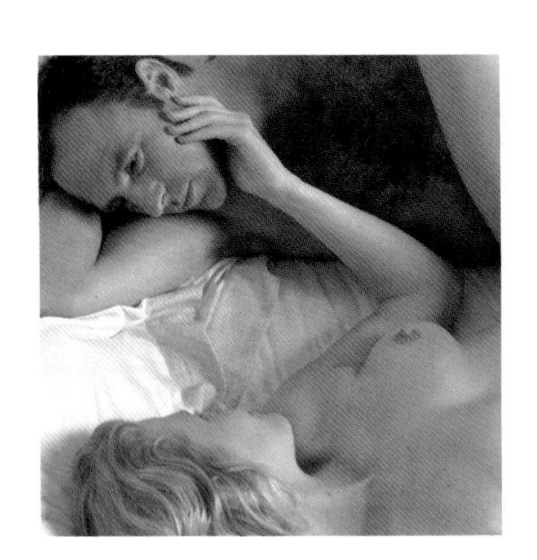

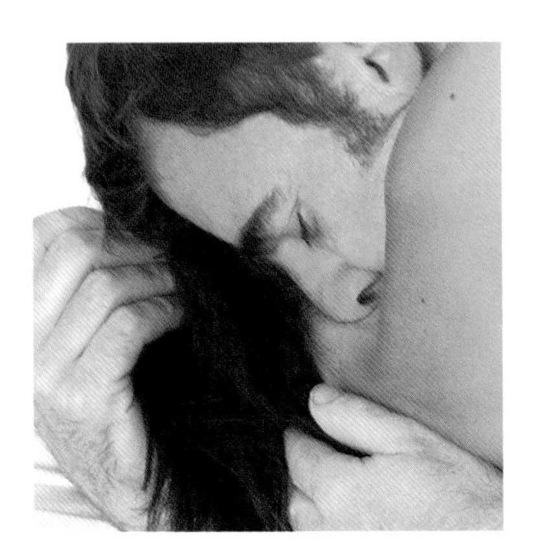

part 4

creative loving

Entering the garden of sensual love, you may feel exhilarated but also lost. Sometimes the garden appears like a tangled mass of leaves, thorns, and flowers, and reaching out to smell the flower, you get pricked by a thorn. The sexual desires and needs of male and female appear to be contradictory, and sexual relations can become awkward.

In this section, the jungle of sexual love is transformed into a garden of delight, as we explore the meaning of Yin and Yang and how to translate this into deeply fulfilling lovemaking for both partners. This exploration has many facets. As you open your eyes to the rainbow of possibilities within sexual union, your garden of love becomes something of timeless beauty. It becomes an ever-deepening exploration, riding the waves of pleasure into the very heart of sexual union, the place where male and female are one circle of bio-electricity. In this circle of energy, you may discover that you are made of the stuff called ecstasy – it is your very nature.

chapter 12

creativity in coitus

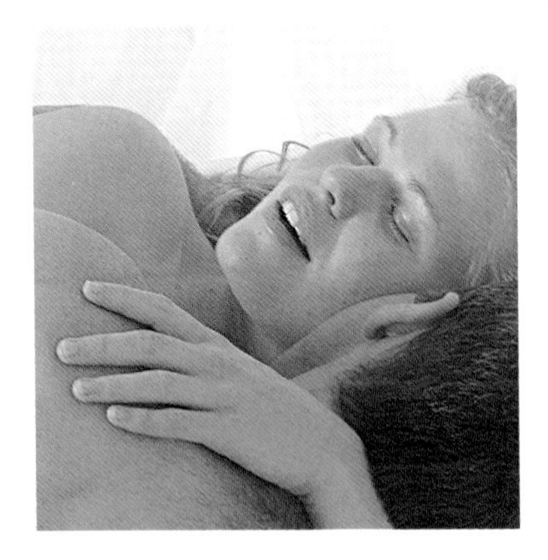

"I will make love with you
But only if you hold me
So my earrings
Touch the jewellery on my ankles"
from a 14th century poem from Arabic Spain

A relationship generally moves along the well-trodden path known as "falling in love". First there is attraction, either sexual or emotional or both. Then follows longing for union, which is often accompanied by burning lust and obsessive fantasy about the love object. Next comes the honeymoon period, which could be as short as one night or could last for several months. There is a tremendous intensity in the surge of sexual hormones, and you are possessed by the need to enter into passionate lovemaking at every opportunity.

"We are both feeling so in love, harmony, and peace together, with a rediscovery of the passion and sexual attraction that we felt when we first met over 10 years ago."

Jivan, Tantra group participant

During the honeymoon period, couples often spontaneously invent all kinds of postures for lovemaking as they glide from one sensorial thrill to another. Gradually they will discover together those postures that seem to offer the most fulfilment within the least amount of time. They then settle down to a routine, which may be satisfying if not earth-shaking for one of the partners, or perhaps both. This intimate partnership may be cosy and nourishing, but lacks the thrill of new discovery. The honeymoon hormones begin to diminish as the cosiness sets in. After about three years the body and mind begin to long for the thrill of the lover's touch that used to sizzle the skin with lust. Many people solve this situation by having secret affairs.

Throughout this scenario, it can be humiliating to realize that you are behaving simply like a puppet on the string of the biological urge to procreate. In this context, "love" is no more than glorified lust. Many people notice how feelings of love swell in them as lust mounts, only to evaporate once genital orgasm has occurred. To be caught in this slavery to very basic biological urges can be depressing. Tantra offers a way of enjoying passionate sex and at the same time nourishing a loving intimacy that is not diminished with time. We call this Rising in Love.

Rising in love

When you rise in love, you are no longer a puppet on the string of biology. Rather, your biology and your mind are both in the service of your higher self, or soul.

This allows space for the soul in sex, or sacred sexuality. When you rise in love, you bring higher wisdom and intelligence to the sex act, lifting it out of mere biological response. The sex act is no longer devoted only to genital release, but becomes a playground where you can discover all the vast potential you have inside – spiritual, mental, emotional, and physical. It becomes a sacred time of experimentation and exploration, expanding you beyond your known limits. You and your lover become pioneers, and sex becomes your voyage of discovery.

There is an old saying that "variety is the spice of life". This is true. And to invite this variety into your love life is a great act of creativity. You become not only a pioneer but an artist, painting your path of love with all the colors of heaven and earth. As you rise in love with your partner, the act of love never becomes routine or boring, no matter how long you have been together. Every day is fresh, virgin with the promise of spring in the air. And each love session is a journey of miraculous discovery.

tips for rising in love

♡ Give priority to nurturing your relationship. Set aside quality time for sexual exploration by making love session appointments with your partner, where you will not be disturbed for at least one hour.

♡ Dare to go into uncharted territory – into positions and places in your intimate sharing where you have not gone before.

♡ Make sure that you both give and receive the types of touch, movements, and tenderness that you need in order to feel complete. Create space for both Yin and Yang styles of lovemaking (see chapter 13).

♡ Appreciate your lover in as many ways as you can – verbally, through touch, in offerings such as a gift or meal, through appreciative eye contact, and by asking her or him what you can do to go deeper into love at this moment.

♡ Experiment with Tantric practices for lovers as a part of your sexual discovery together.

creating the ambience for thrilling lovemaking

♡ Write a list of all the things that turn you on and give you the thrill of a new love affair.

♡ Draw on your experience of past and present love affairs, thinking of things that used to excite you and things that still do.

♡ Include even the most intimate ways your partner used to touch you, or look at you.

♡ What kinds of activities do you find erotic or thrilling? Perhaps you like to watch your partner undress, or you adore being kissed on the neck, or you love the scent of your partner after exercise, or it drives you wild to hear sensual words whispered in your ear.

♡ Make a date with your partner. During the date you should both consciously create the ambience for one or more of the thrilling experiences from your list. You may have to explain carefully to your lover what is needed. Your partner is not taking on the personality of a past lover, but simply supporting you in creating a tried and tested way of being that turns you on.

♡ Take turns to be the one who asks for the ambience to inspire the thrill. Make up your own schedule of dates. Perhaps one weekend it is your turn and the next weekend it is your lover's turn. Just be careful to make it a two-way street – each of you should have the same number of turns at this.

a meditation for rising in love

♡ Choose a room with enough space for you to move across it. Soften the lighting and put on some soulful music.

♡ Stand facing each other on opposite sides of the room, either naked or lightly clothed. Gaze into each other's eyes as you start to move slowly toward each other. Feel the nuances and different qualities of each millimetre as you approach each other slowly but surely through the layers of your auras. This slow approach could take as long as 15 minutes.

♡ When your bellies are barely touching, close your eyes. Raise your arms into the air and silently request cosmic energy to fill your body and move you into the type of love union it wishes.

♡ Surrender totally to this mysterious energy. You are being moved by a superior force not born of your will. Simply let go of all doing, and be possessed by divine energy.

♡ Trust in the flow as you undulate together, mingling bodies and souls. Be in a state of not knowing. Let each moment bring a fresh surprise. This type of love union may or may not come to penetrative sex. It may or may not come to orgasm. Just trust what wants to happen from your higher self.

♡ Throughout this whole experience allow sounds to come, but do not talk since this leaks energy away from the delicate and transformative spaces you are moving into.

♡ When your love session feels complete, Namaste each other. Namaste means "I bow down to the divine within you". Hold your hands together as for praying, in front of your chest, and look into your lover's eyes as you bow slightly from the waist.

playing with different positions

When you play with different positions during lovemaking you invite a whole spectrum of qualities into your love relating. Each posture will activate a different kind of response. The more expansive you can be with how you express your love, and the more dimensions you can include, the more spicy and fulfilling your relating will be. Instead of being one-dimensional, always moving into the same habits of behavior, you will become multi-dimensional – able to access new and unexpected facets of your being. This will help you to open to new experiences and qualities in lovemaking. You will be challenged to open up more of your potential, not only as lovers but as individuals.

The photographs on pages 101–105 illustrate 13 basic sexual postures. There are also many variations on these. Allow yourselves to flow into new positions out of your spontaneous creativity.

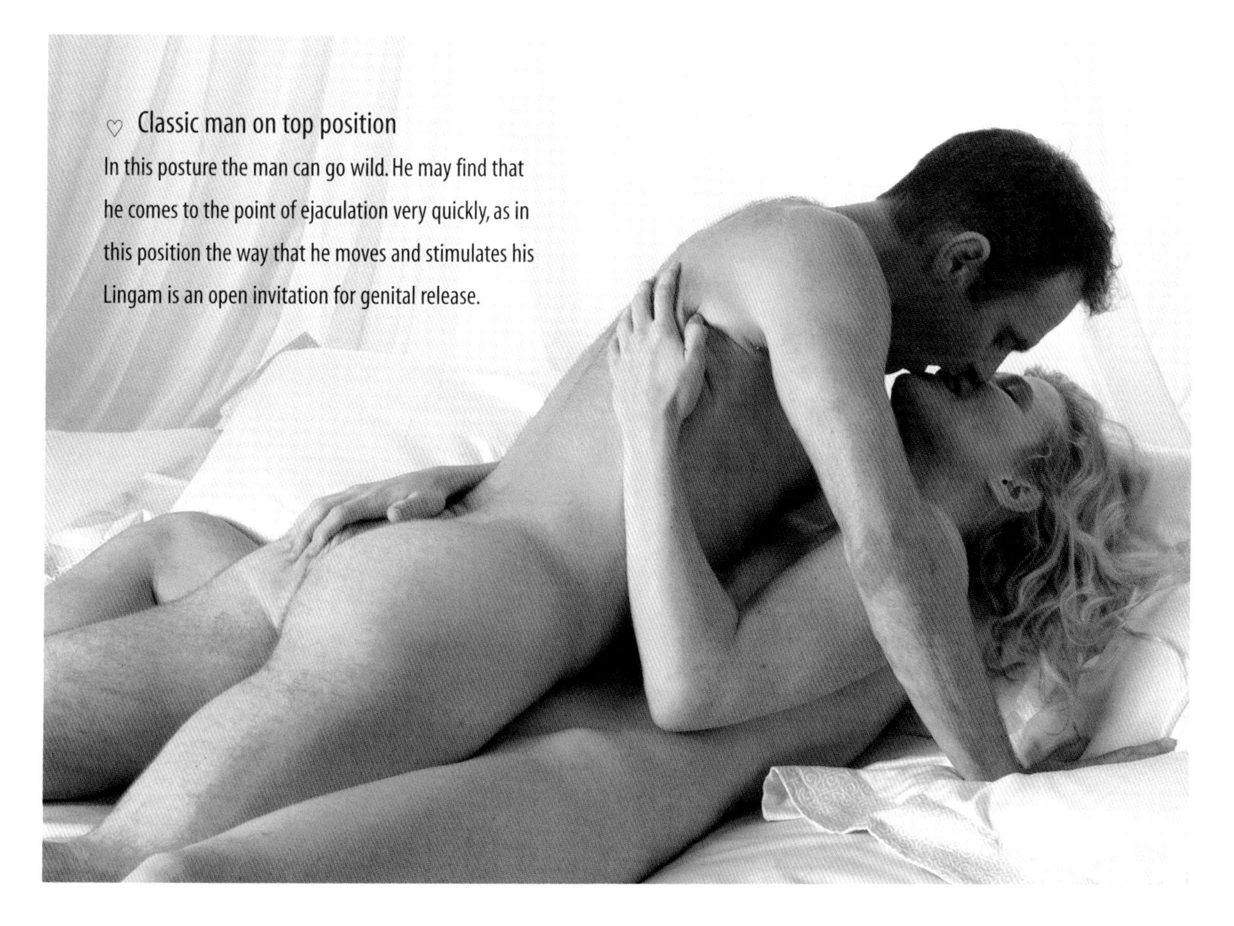

♡ Classic man on top position

In this posture the man can go wild. He may find that he comes to the point of ejaculation very quickly, as in this position the way that he moves and stimulates his Lingam is an open invitation for genital release.

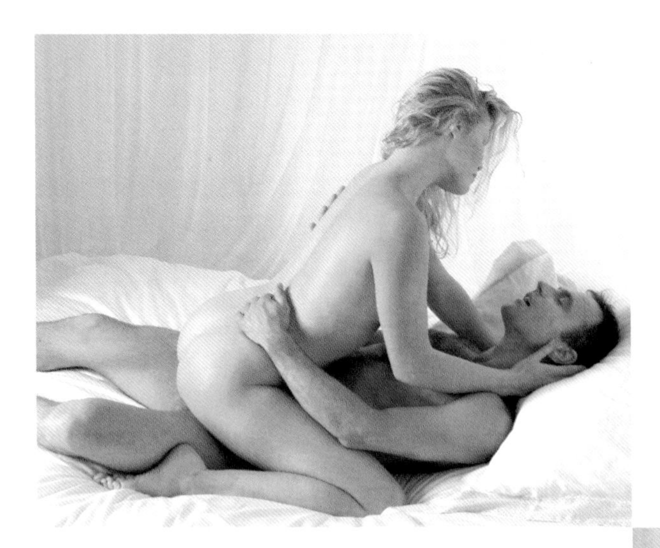

♡ Woman on top

In this posture the woman can go wild. It is a good position to bring a woman to orgasm, as she is able to stimulate her clitoris through her body movements.

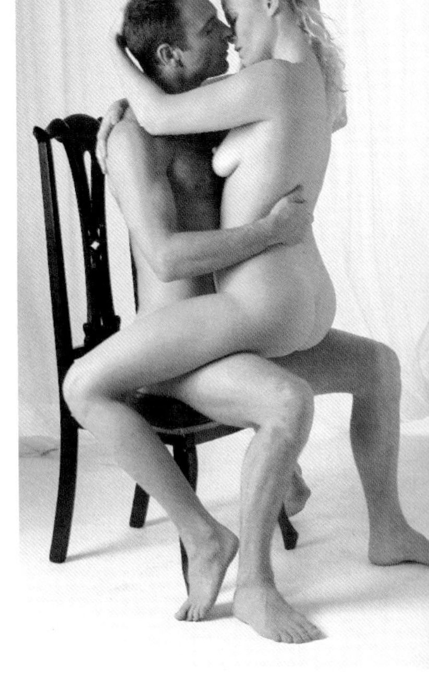

♡ Throne position

This is a relaxing way to be a king and queen of love, sitting together in a chair with the woman on top. It allows for a very pleasurable rocking motion, deep penetration, and stimulation of the woman's clitoris through her movements.

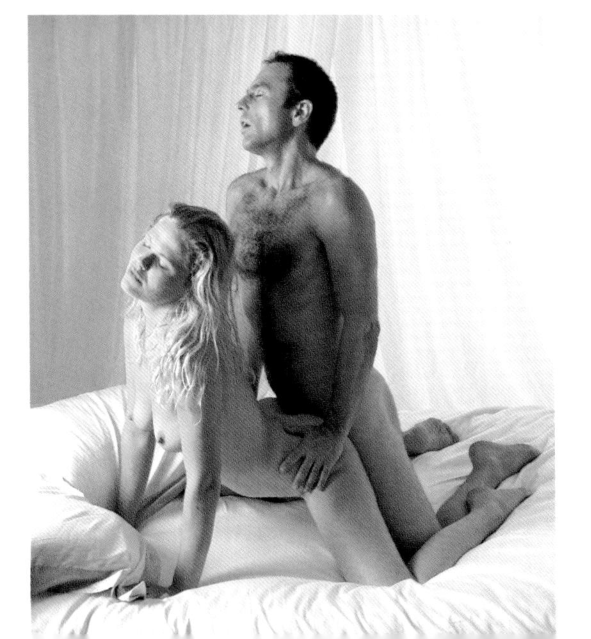

♡ Lion position

In this posture the man enters the woman's Yoni from behind, allowing for deep penetration and letting the woman feel totally possessed by her mate. For an additional rush of pleasure, the man can bite the back of his lover's neck. For this position the woman needs to be fully ready and wet, with her Yoni in full arousal.

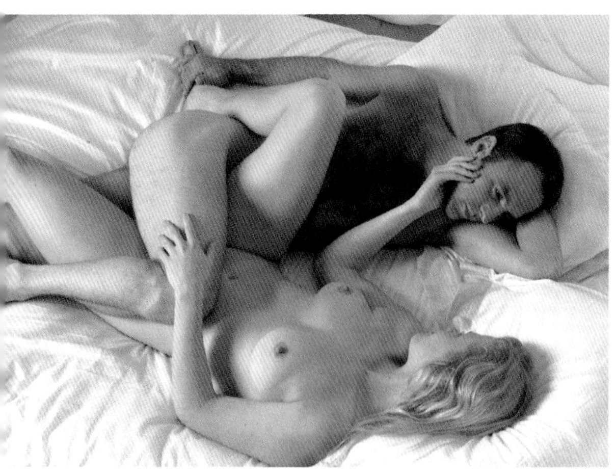

♡ Scissors position

This posture allows the man and woman to relax together in the space of valley orgasm (see page 117). In this position the woman can insert a non-erect Lingam into her Yoni. This "plugging in" allows the couple to enter into deep intimacy and helps the woman to expand in her feminine nature, since it is a Yin position (see page 109). Rest in this state for at least 20 minutes to experience its full benefit.

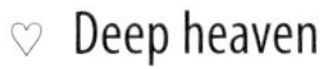

♡ Deep heaven

This position is easy to slide into from the Scissors. It allows for soft movements deep inside the Yoni, which are relaxing, nourishing, and uplifting. Try just being still when you reach the pleasure zone and experience heaven on earth.

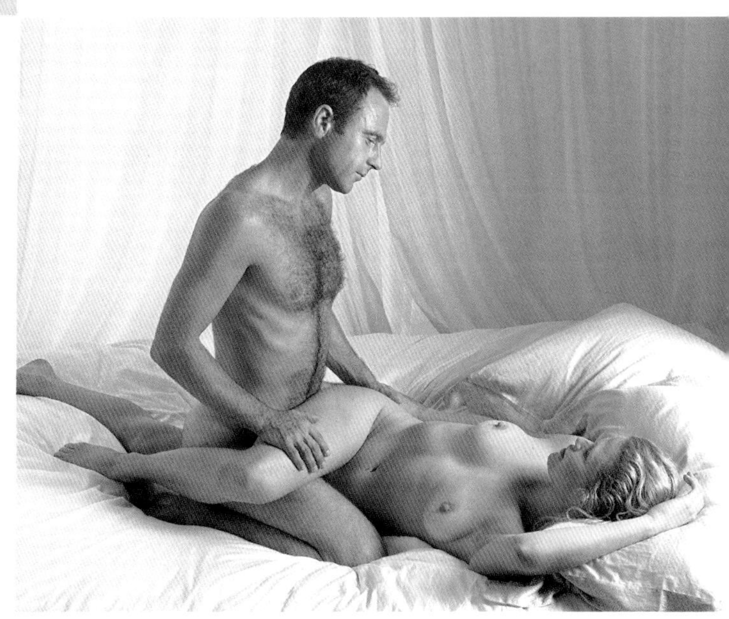

♡ Yab Yum

The classic Tantra Position. This posture encourages the merging of all seven chakras (see page 78), joining sexual energy with superconsciousness. Try putting your foreheads together and breathing in unison to bring about an opening of the third eye.

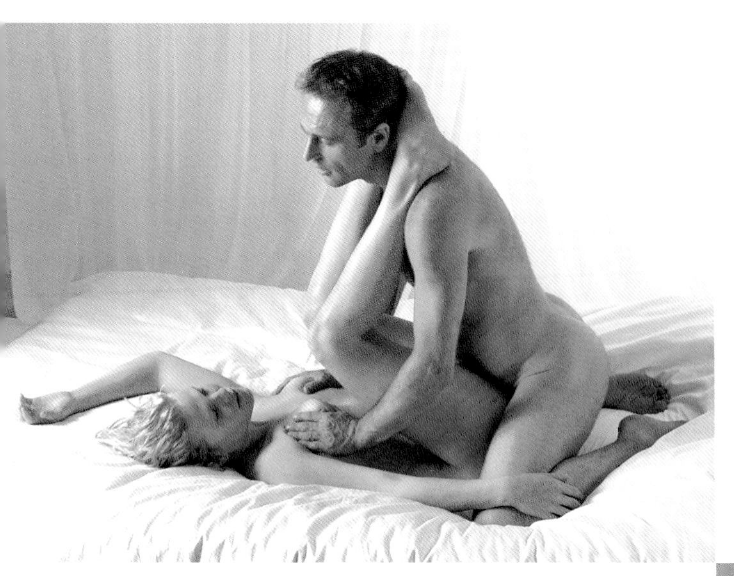

♡ The plough

When used in lovemaking, this yoga posture is an ideal position for the man to plant his seed in the womb of his earth goddess. The posture allows for deep penetration, but be careful, as the Yoni is stretched and may be sensitive.

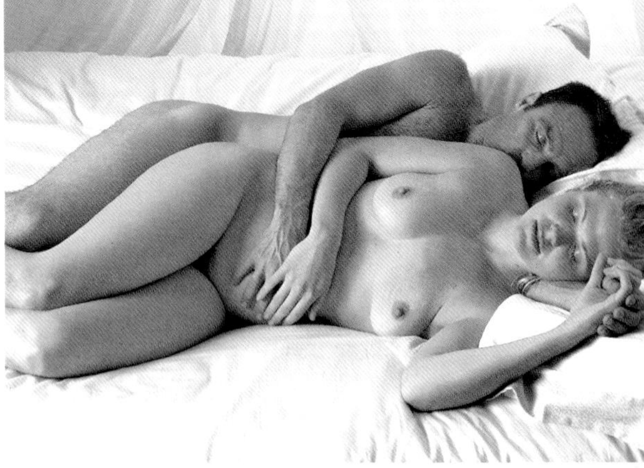

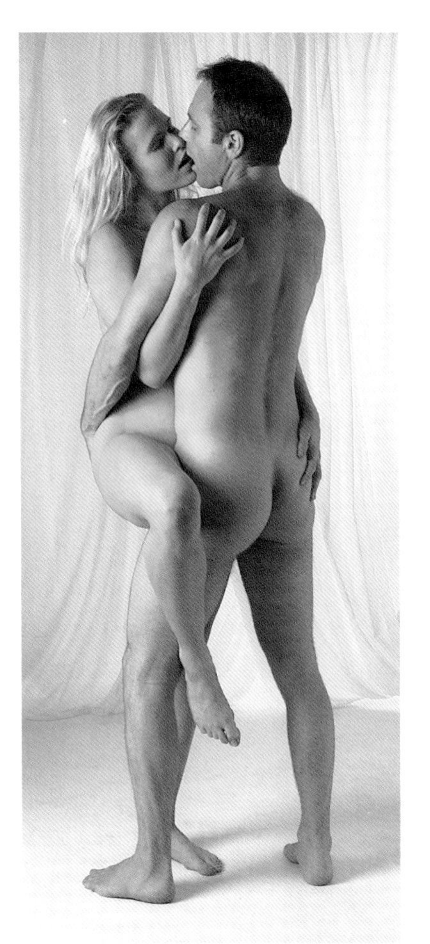

♡ Spooning

This is a comfort position, especially good for falling asleep together. The man's arm surrounds the woman and rests on her belly, as he relaxes with his Lingam inside her Yoni from behind.

♡ Standing position

This position can be used almost anytime, anywhere when the heat of the moment is upon you – in the forest against a tree, for example. The man can enter the woman's Yoni either from in front or from behind.

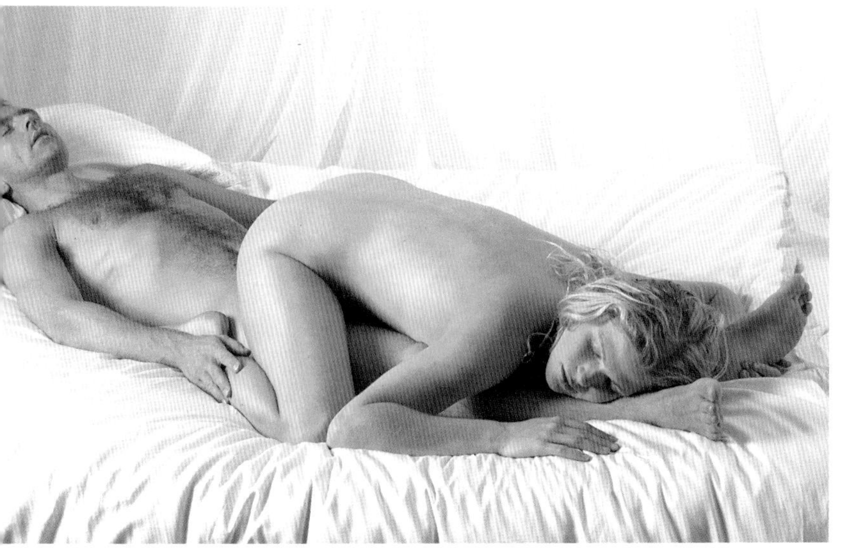

♡ Recharging position

A magical position for recharging your energy after making love for a while. The woman sits astride her partner, with his Lingam inside her, facing his feet. Then she slowly bends over until her head rests at his feet. When you are both comfortable, lie still and recharge for 10 minutes or more.

♡ Woman's delight

The woman sits on the man's erect Lingam with her back toward his chest, leaning back against him. Her legs are open wide and she relaxes completely. The man is then free to play with her breasts and clitoris with his hands, teasing her slowly into complete arousal. The man cannot move easily, so the woman may wish to swivel her hips a little from time to time, just enough to maintain his erection. In this position the woman can allow her own arousal without feeling overpowered by the man's movements.

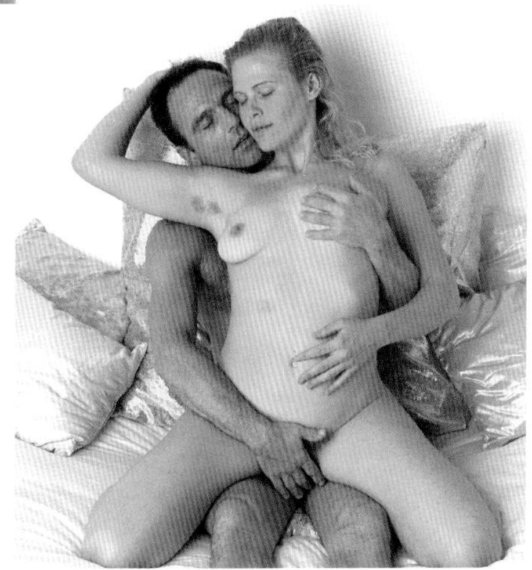

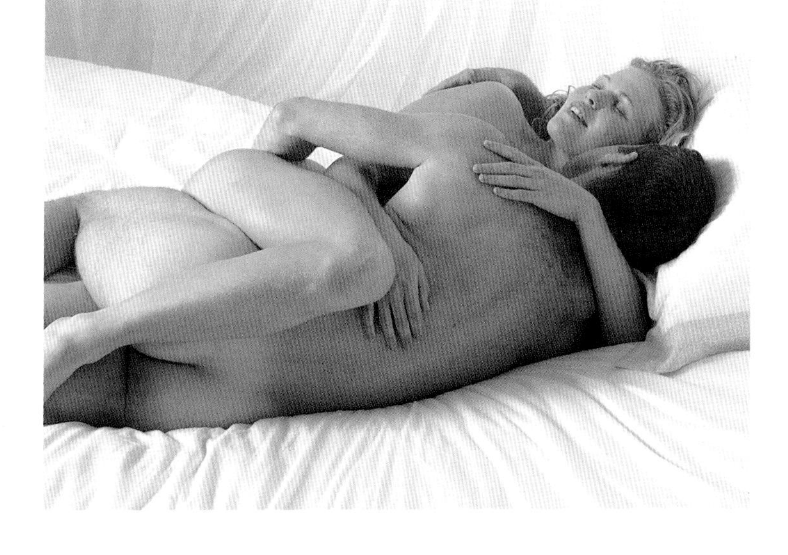

♡ Lovers' embrace

This is a very easy and natural position for lovemaking. Both partners can melt into each other, moving or being still, relaxed or passionate as the mood indicates. The position allows one or both partners to play with the woman's clitoris during penetration, and to be able to kiss and fondle each other easily. The leg positions can be changed according to what feels most comfortable for both partners.

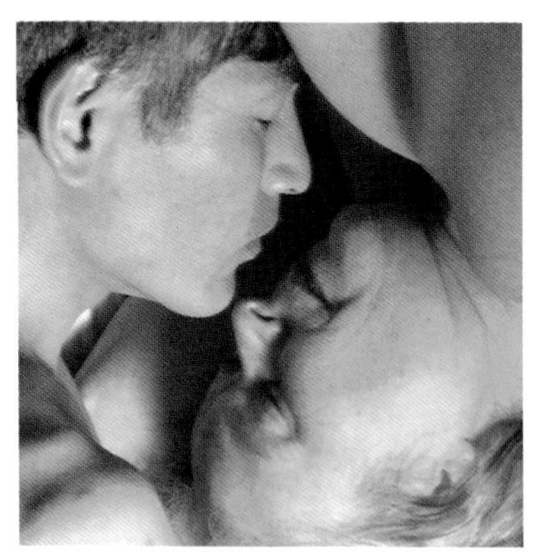

sex act in Yin, sex act in Yang

"The valley spirit never dies
It is named the mysterious female
And the doorway of the mysterious female
Is the base from which heaven and earth spring
It is there within us all the while
Draw upon it as you will
It never runs dry"
Tao Te Ching, Lao Tzu, China, 6th century BC

A woman with her lover, in general, loves to cuddle, whisper sweet nothings, caress and be caressed, taking all the time in the world simply to be, losing herself in that space beyond time and mind where love rules. Generally, women never get enough of this type of interaction with their male partners. Women often complain "Why can't a man be romantic, or cuddly?" Many women say that their favourite part of sex is the holding and cuddling. However, because women have an idea that their sexuality should be like a man's, they may not accept their need to be soft and cuddly. So they deny this part of themselves and are thus many times unfulfilled, taking their revenge by being bitchy and nagging.

When a man and woman make love it is a meeting of two diametrically opposite aspects. If the woman can accept her nature and celebrate it, she will become a great teacher for the man. To be balanced in himself, he needs what the woman has; that is why there is attraction. But he cannot get it if the woman denies and represses that feminine quality in herself. Women need to really be themselves in sex and take the space they need.

The male lover goes for strong Yang activity during sex. The female needs to balance this with her capacity to sink deep into Yin, an abyss of love and restfulness, just holding each other and diving deeper and deeper into the unknown. In Tantra, this state is called the valley orgasm (see page 117). The higher the peak, the deeper the valley. And the deeper the valley, the higher the peak. They go hand in hand. If you have only fiery activity in sex you will miss the depths of love. The woman is the teacher of the valley orgasm for the man. And the man is the teacher of the peak orgasm for the woman. But first the woman needs to explore and accept her nature. When she has totally embraced her Yin, then she will also be able to discover her capacity for Yang passion within herself.

Making love in Yin

The method of making love in Yin (see page 109) was first described by a Chinese physician, Master Sun, and has since been "rediscovered" several times over the centuries. It is based on relaxation and non-doing. Arousal is allowed, but not from a place of activity. It is a happening, like waves in the ocean that rise up and then melt back. The method is very nourishing for the woman and regenerating for the man, and offers space for a couple to dive deep into the experience of the valley orgasm.

On the spiritual path, which is synonymous with the path of sex and love, a woman's way is the way of devotion. However, she also carries the opposite characteristics: she can be fiery, passionate, and ruthless. Her tremendous power, which has masculine characteristics, is only seen once she has dived deeply into her devotional nature, so deep that she encounters the opposite and complementary aspect of herself and thus becomes whole. If the woman accepts her Yin nature during sex, during that same love session she will connect with tremendous sources of fire and passion she may never have known she possessed. She will become absolutely wild. Her ecstasy will know no limits.

You may think that if the goal is for a woman to manifest her complementary opposite, she can work to cultivate this. But remember that anything cultivated is not natural – it is something artificial imposed on nature. It will not bring the same results and deep satisfaction. Truth is found by embracing who you are as deeply as you can. When you have achieved that, then and only then will the real and precious flower of your total potential be revealed to you. It will happen without any effort. It is all a question of letting go into your own nature. This applies equally to sex, love, and spirituality. A woman needs to know and understand the laws of Yin, to know herself as the abyss, the unfathomable mystery, the womb, and to let this guide her into the very heart of love.

"Before I was with Sarita I experimented with this method with various partners and found it very valuable. One of the benefits I got from it was the understanding and experience of how energies get connected with a woman, that it is not a question of effort but more of a let go, a trust in the body. It has given me the understanding that tuning into myself is the way to tune into my partner, as well as being a way to discover more subtle aspects of sexual energies. Before that, I had never really experienced how waves of energy happen of their own accord and that it was up to me just to allow them to move my body or to bring me to stillness. Those experiences helped to transform my life and my experience of sexuality."

Geho

The way of Yin

The great Taoist master Lao Tzu said that "water wears away rock". In the same way Yin, though apparently weaker and more fragile than Yang, is actually more powerful. This law of life gives the woman patience, even if she has never thought about it. A woman teaches the way of Yin in a thousand small ways in everyday life, just like water slowly eroding the rock of apparent reality. In her relationships she will often find her way through a dilemma simply by remaining silent, or by saying "Yes" to the man and then waiting for the inevitable, which her intuition told her was the right direction. She yields, and in her yielding the truth of a situation becomes apparent.

This quality brings dignity and grace to the woman. If she can tune into this watery, yielding aspect of herself she will discover a tremendous inner strength. She will keep moving in the direction she is attuned to, no matter what may come. If you look at a river, the rocks and boulders offer a challenge to the water, which responds by forming rapids or waterfalls, awesome and powerful in their effect. Remember this power so that you do not make the mistake of thinking Yin means yielding, equalling weak or inferior. Yin is simply a different sort of power to the man's Yang.

We can consider women's same-sex relationships in the same terms. There is another Taoist observation that water coming from two sources merges together naturally and easily. Both Indian and Taoist Tantra traditions believe that women merging and melting one with the other are not creating a harmful effect but rather a natural one. Love play between women is simply nourishing them to expand their Yin qualities of love, devotion, softness, and melting.

However, this does not mean that lesbianism is preferable to heterosexuality. If a woman makes love exclusively to other women she misses the great benefit and teaching that will come to her through merging with the opposite sex. The current trend, where heterosexual women also occasionally make love with girlfriends, is healthy and natural. Although not every woman needs this, it can be celebrated as an affirmation of femininity.

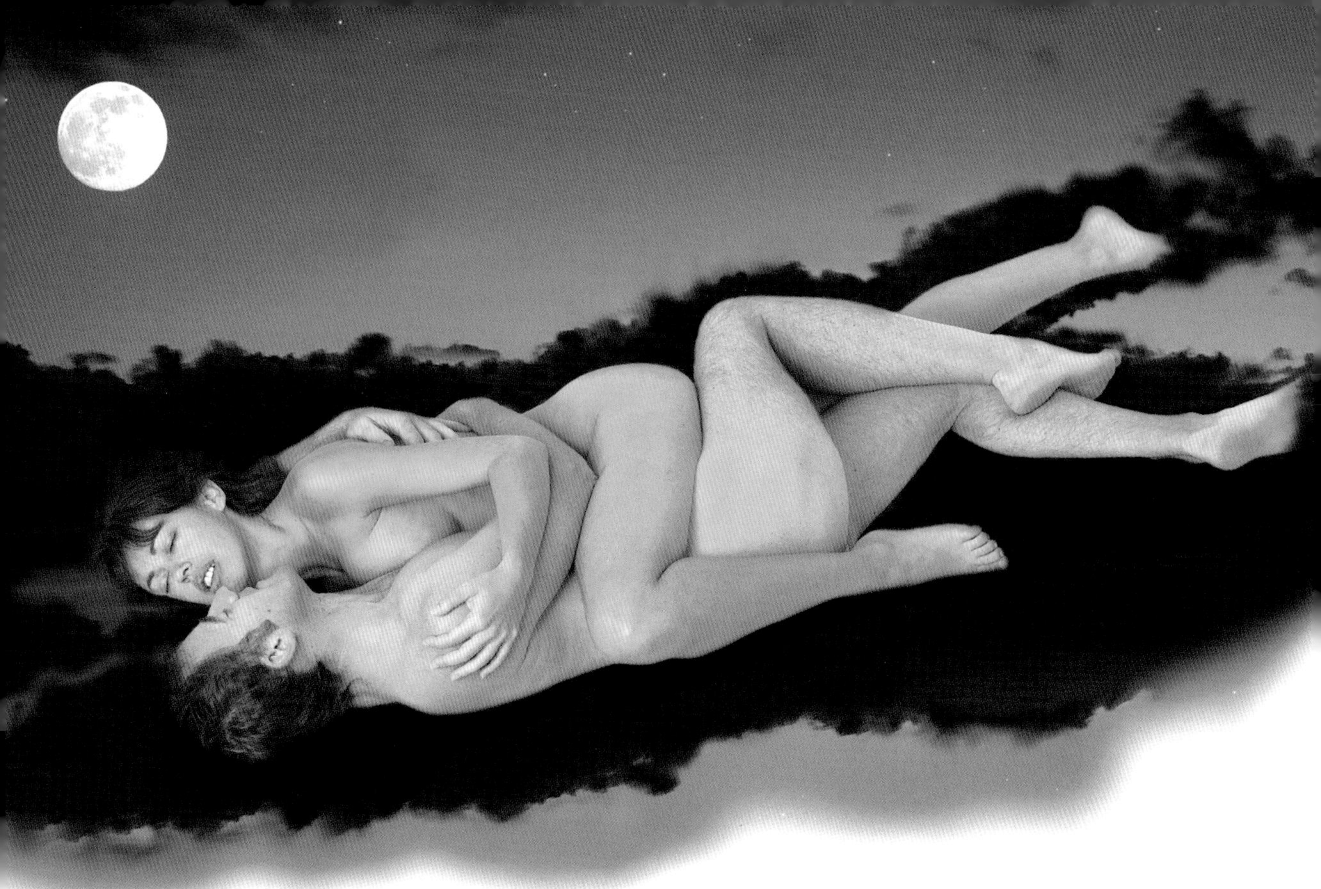

how to make love in Yin

Just lying with your partner, present but in a space of non-doing, something starts to happen, a meeting and exchange of energy. This method deepens intimacy and helps you both to become more familiar with Yin spaces in your lovemaking.

♡ Lie on your side facing each other, on either side of the bed, looking into each other's eyes. Move a little closer in small steps, taking time to relax all tensions. Each time you move closer, tune into your body and find out how it is to connect with your partner at that distance. There is no rush for the bodies to meet; this process of tuning in to yourself and your partner can take at least 20 minutes.

♡ Finally come into contact with your partner's body. Just relax, do nothing, not even caressing or moving the body voluntarily. After some moments, if the man has an erection or half an erection, it is time for penetration. The scissors position is best (see page 103). If he has no erection, penetration is still possible. The woman can slowly pull back the man's foreskin and using two fingers just above the crown of the Lingam and two fingers of her other hand at the base, she can gently push the Lingam into her Yoni, a little at a time.

♡ Once the Lingam is inside the Yoni, simply wait and find out what wants to happen. The body may move of its own accord, but do not provoke movements yourself. Waves of energy may take your body into movements of ecstasy, but always come back to relaxation and non-doing. Erections come and go – allow this to happen. Stay plugged in like this for at least 40 minutes.

Whenever you feel attracted to a particular method of lovemaking it is wise to go into it in a series of love appointments of agreed duration. When you have completed the commitment, let go of the structure and be simple and natural. In this way you will always be able to find a balance.

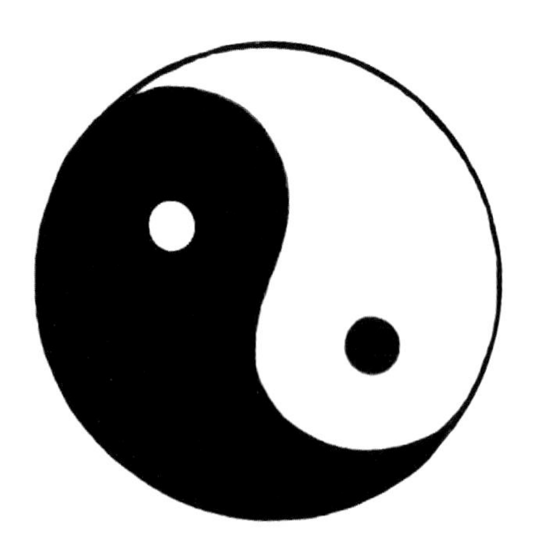

Yin and Yang

The Yin Yang symbol, created in ancient China, contains all that is valuable in the great religious teachings of the world, and an essential life lesson. In addition, it carries potent teaching on the nature of sexual relations between man and woman.

The black area symbolizes the female, Yin quality of existence, which can be said to encompass the cool, resting, flowing, yielding, and receptive aspects of life. The white area symbolizes the male, Yang qualities, encompassing the hot, active, hard, strong, outgoing aspects of life. The black and white areas are cocooned into each other, much as a man and woman may lie in each other's arms. The black contains a small circle of white, while the white has a small circle of black, indicating that Yin moves into Yang, and Yang moves into Yin.

In lovemaking, as you let go deeply into the Yin, resting state, you will automatically find yourself entering the Yang, outgoing state. Likewise, if you go totally into the active Yang state, you will automatically move into the Yin, resting state. Life always seeks balance, through a flow between Yin and Yang.

The examples of this universal law are all around us. Each breath consists of a Yin, letting go, out-breath followed by a Yang, life-regenerating, in-breath, each one cocooned into the next in an undulating wave. You go to sleep (Yin) and you wake up (Yang). Night (Yin) gives way to day and day (Yang) to night. You are man or woman but you also contain the qualities of the opposite sex.

When a person attains to an expansive state of consciousness, the realization comes that wherever contradictions of life meet, there you will find the ultimate truth. The mind tends to want to grasp only one aspect of life. The Yin Yang symbol is a clear reminder to embrace opposite, complementary polarities, for it is there, in that place of meeting, that you will know the very essence of life.

A perfectly balanced man is able to be both passionate and sensitive. He knows how to live both the state of Yang and the state of Yin, expanding his consciousness to include the whole of what life has to offer. A perfectly balanced woman is able to be yielding, receptive, and loving, as well as powerfully forthright.

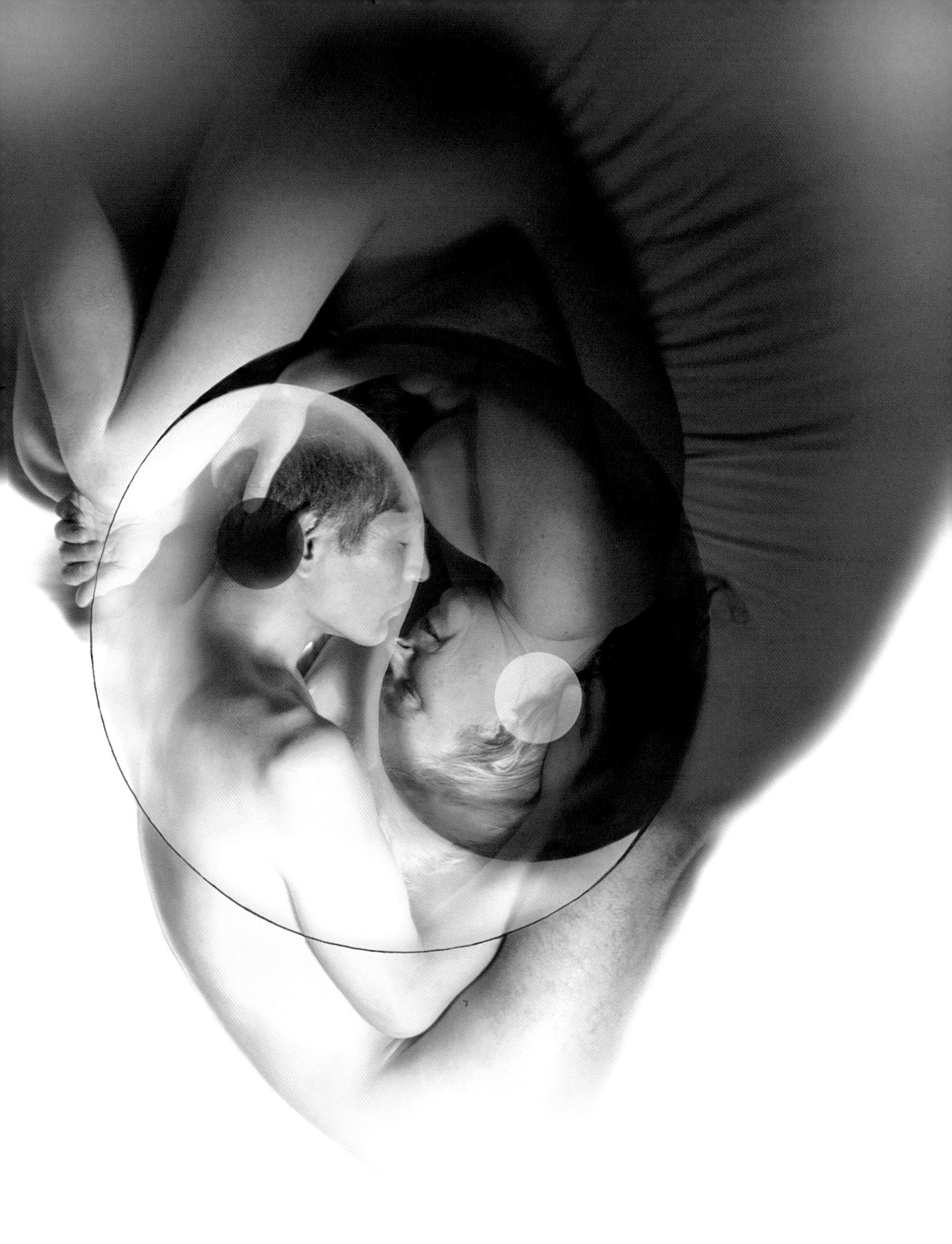

Male creative energies

"When in such embrace your senses are shaken as leaves, enter this shaking."

Shiva Sutra

Male energy is a penetrative, powerful, creative force and its nature is to seek expression. This energy is fiery, hot, active, emissive, decisive, expressive, strong, straight, initiative, exciting, igniting, rising, radiant, and luminous. When male energy is at play in its pure form, all these miraculous qualities are present, enlightening the world. However because of its outgoing nature, male energy tends to start seeking something "out there", outside itself, sometimes getting lost and unable to find its way home. Female energy is always "down to earth", and the woman brings the man back to a balanced experience of life.

Male energy is daring and moves toward new discoveries and goals, whether spiritual or material. Seeking itself, it goes on a search for new spaces of being, or things that reflect the mystery of creation. Since the beginning of time, man has used his energy for developing objects, devices, and inventions, as well as in the arts, in an effort to embellish and improve his outer life. The evolution of his mind has brought him freedom to think and to create the kind of lifestyle he thinks will be best. However, he frequently gets lost in his disconnected world, and wastes his energy in directions and projects that prove destructive or out of tune with life's principles. When this happens, it is a sign that he is ignoring the soul dimension of his energy.

The same principles apply to sexuality. In sex, a man tends to get stuck into a groove that he follows. This may be right at first, but he becomes blind to how the energy has already shifted, or wants to shift. The man finds himself in a dilemma: whether to follow or control his instinctual impulses. Only a man could ask the question: To be or not to be? The question would not enter a woman's mind. He is uncertain of his role in the creation of life. The macho or hard man tries to hide his shakiness by playing a role that every woman knows is just a put-on.

Merging instinct and consciousness

Basic instinctual behaviors are programmed by nature. These aspects of man have been much condemned by societies and religions and the so-called "civilized" man has some level of shame around them. The effort to repress male instinct, where male energy is rooted, has brought countless perversions into the world. If energy has no natural outlet, it will find perverted ways of expression. Sexual perversions, the "mental sexuality" prevalent in our society, and violence, fanaticism, a sense of being lost and not knowing the "meaning of life" are all examples of this. Either a man accepts his raw instinct, or he is a man without roots – and without roots a plant cannot grow or flower. The man's personal and spiritual development depend on how he can accept, live, and play with his basic instinctual energy.

If the man can turn his outgoing creative power inward, he will awaken his consciousness and be in tune with the calling of his soul and his divine nature. Only then can the outer expression of his energy be in tune with the highest principles. Consciousness is the key in harnessing a man's creative powers and allowing him to reach his full potential as a co-creator of life. It allows him to expand beyond the body and mind into new levels of bliss and ecstasy, beyond a one-dimensional, instinctual way of being.

Some men reject their instinctual nature and try to prove themselves "above" it, using the mind, logical rationalizations, philosophies, scholarly studies, and theories. They believe that it is this logic that raises man above the animal kingdom. The mind is an amazing bio-computer, a beautiful tool that serves intelligence, but it is very much bound to the body, the instinctual nature, the conditioning of society and the environment. The mind itself is not intelligent. If you ask it to stop thinking, it does not – it goes on like a broken record.

Where there is consciousness, the thinking mechanism has a more refined quality of true intelligence, a quality of witnessing, with an overview of the body, mind, and emotions. This true intelligence can be brought forward from the soul level, through Tantric meditation.

When consciousness arising from the soul level merges with instinctual qualities, the result is a celebration of life energy within the context of love and a respectful attitude toward all of life. Matter is infused with the light of the spirit; the instinctual becomes illumined and simultaneously ennobled.

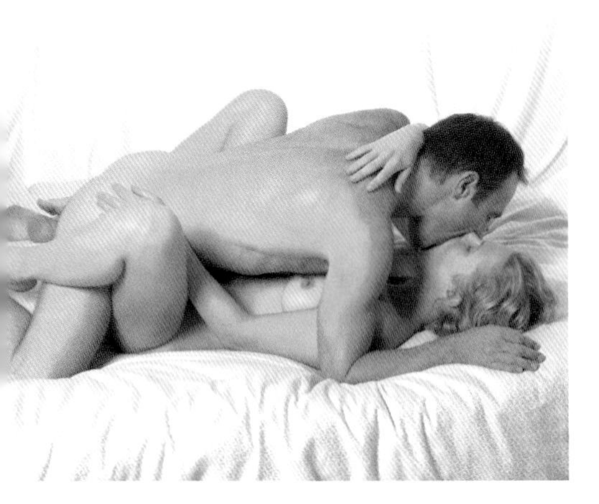

Making love in Yang

Tantra is conscious of the whole of man and denies nothing. It works with a man's instinctual aspects, and transforms them into a nectar of fulfilment. In sex, the fiery and wild nature of male energy takes the couple into an exalted state of being: a peak experience. In order to know this experience, the couple have to allow their wildness in its pure form, with a total let go into passion. This is an experience of pure, untamed energy, streaming all over the body, leaving no part that is not orgasmic. The localized genital experience of sexuality gets transformed into a whole-body orgasmic experience.

To attain whole-body orgasm, the man needs to allow his whole body to become the Lingam, and the woman to allow her whole body to be the Yoni. The couple will lose their sense of self and become pure energy. Then they can live passion in its fullest form and the man can be multi-orgasmic. This pure form of passion is more than just the man thrusting strongly, provoking a hot moment of intensity that leads quickly to ejaculation. That is not enough to unleash the incredible gifts contained in the male spark. The body needs to be allowed to move in many more ways than just "thrusting". The energy of passion itself will move the body uncontrollably.

Sounds are also very important. Allow yourself to make all kinds of sounds, without censoring them. Without sounds, you cannot have a truly passionate experience. Forget all about "civilization". Return to your wild animal state.

Allowing yourself to live your Yang passionate energy will free you from restrictive ways of sexual relating. Knowing the wild man in yourself will also make you very attractive to women. A woman searches for a man of passion, for only with such a man can she discover her own totality in orgasm through her wild Yang aspect.

Tantricas in India have always been wild and untamed people, because they know that the great existential laws are not bound to what we call "civilization". They practice wild, ecstatic dancing, because it is a very potent way of opening the body and energy to new expanded states of being. Through dancing they reach a trance-like state, where they disappear as a self and only Shiva is. In that moment, the dancer is elevated to the realm of the gods.

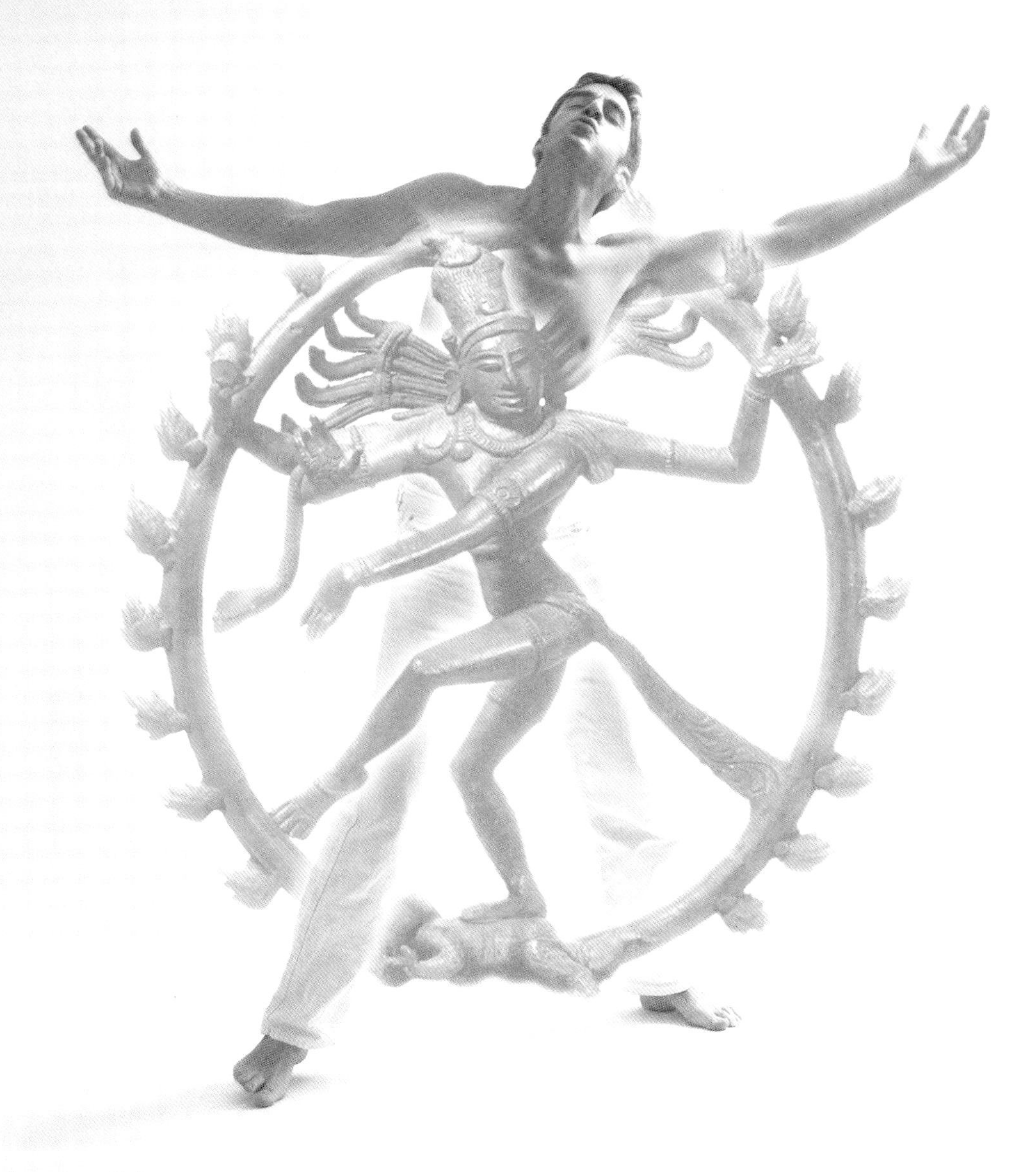

Nataraj: the dancing Shiva

Nataraj, which means "Lord of the Dance", is one of the names of Shiva, who created the world through dance. Both men and women can practice this meditation. Entering totally into the experience of both phases will bring balance, helping Yin and Yang to merge inside you.

♡ Yang phase: Dance ecstatically for 40 minutes. Become the Shiva Linga, dancing the stars, the sun and the moon, the trees and the plants, the mountains and the sky, and the animals. Become one with the power that creates the whole of life.

♡ Yin phase: Lie down for 15 minutes in complete stillness and let go.

♡ Get up and dance again softly for 3 minutes, bringing integration.

For a CD to accompany this meditation, see Resources, page 189.

chapter 14

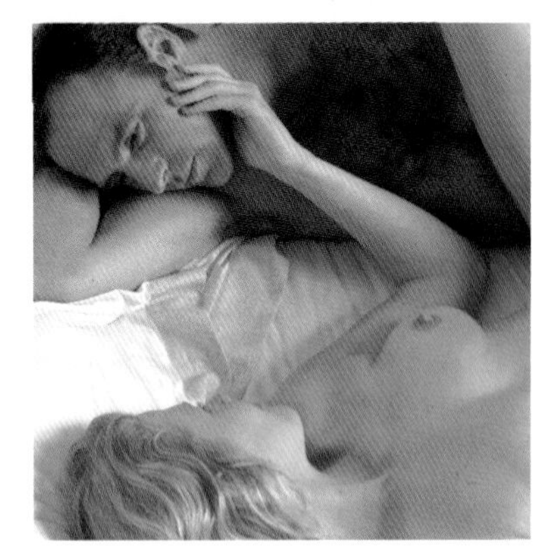

fulfilled sex in partnership

"Heaven (male) creates, earth (female) is receptive
The male is active, and so seeks stillness
The female is still, and so seeks activity
Each must acquire the essence of the other
To be complete"
White Tigress Manual, Female Taoist Masters, China, 18th century, translated by Hsi Lai

For fulfilling sex, both the man and the woman need equal space to express and experience their unique qualities. Just as the sun and moon both need their time to shine during a 24-hour cycle, so it is with man and woman during a cycle of lovemaking. The diagram shows a series of three peaks and three valleys, each one moving successively higher or deeper. These represent the cycles of Yang moving into Yin in undulating waves during a love session. These cycles of Yin and Yang cannot be produced through a technique; this natural phenomenon occurs on its own every time you make love. So to experience fulfilment, you simply need to allow what happens naturally.

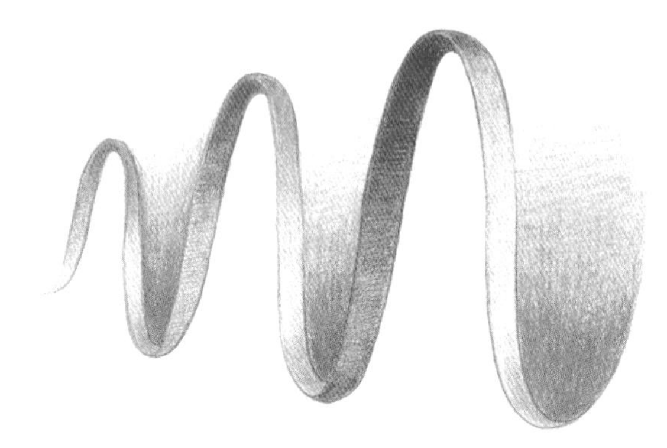

Because most people are not educated in the sensual arts, sex is generally viewed as the domain of Yang, peak arousal. A couple get together with the goal of orgasm reverberating inside, with a feverish intensity, like a hot fire that is soon extinguished. The woman tries to match the man's heat and excitement as best she can. The couple then move into passionate sex, designed to reach quickly a state of Yang or male climax. The sex act is then considered to be finished. If the woman is lucky in this scenario, she will have managed to climb the mountain of excitement as quickly as her lover does. Many women are not able to do this so quickly, and they simply give up and fake orgasm or pretend that their orgasm doesn't matter.

There is nothing wrong with "peak" sex. However if this is the only way a couple makes love, it is limited and does not allow the feminine energy to expand.

exploring the peaks and valleys of love

If we bring awareness to sex, we may find a very different scenario, as described below. Awareness means simply witnessing and going with what is, without allowing the mind to judge and control.

The couple wants sex. She craves physical tenderness and a slow build-up; he wants penetration. She initiates tenderness by lovingly caressing and stroking him, including the place that is all heated up in him – his Lingam. She speaks words of appreciation for the wonder of this beautiful god as she caresses and massages him there, not to turn him on, but to open a fluidity of sensual energy that she then spreads all over by caressing his whole body. He feels nourished, more relaxed, and awakens to the wonders of sensual appreciative touch.

He caresses her body, focusing on the lower belly, to help her open sexually. The touch is relaxed, not trying to turn her on, but loving and appreciating her goddess nature. Then he moves to her breasts, loving her there with caressing, massage, and appreciative words. His caresses then spread this awakened energy all over her body.

Now that her basic need has been fulfilled they start kissing passionately. He touches her Yoni, and finding it swollen and juicy, he goes on touching her there, or honors her Yoni by kissing it. When she is longing for penetration, he enters her. They begin moving toward a peak, enjoying the intense pleasure. They start feeling fused, as if they have become one pillar of energy. But then, before the call for ejaculation whispers, there is a "gap", where one or both suddenly feel detached, the heat of passion suddenly drops. This delicate space can be missed. The man might think something is "wrong" and go on trying to keep the energy moving toward a higher peak. If he relaxes into the gap, his erection may soften. Relaxation steals over both of them. The soft Lingam may even come out of the Yoni.

This is where Yin takes possession of them. They relax as one, deep in the valley of love. They remain unmoving, still fused, yet utterly relaxed, breathing in unison, with slow, deep breaths. They may place their third eye centers together, bringing them into utter absorption, an oceanic no-mind state. They lie like this for perhaps 15 minutes, in a space of deep meditation. Then, mysteriously, they slowly emerge from the cool depth of the ocean. The desire to express love is coming back. A subtle heat surrounds them, they feel excitement and new pleasure building up. They begin to explore each other's bodies anew.

This time as they begin ascending the peak, they are more free, more joyous, and more in love than ever before. New sources of energy have been unleashed, which seem to have no limits. In this second ascent toward the peak the woman has had time to expand into her Yin nature, so she is relaxed and in tune with her partner. Male and female are equally matched. A quality of timeless exquisite bliss infuses them both. A yearning to go on infinitely in this space may slow their movements, leading them softly into a second valley. There they remain, suffused in ecstatic oneness of body and soul. This ascent, and the valley that follows may each take 15–20 minutes.

By the third peak, they have become drunk on the divine play of love. They are one circle of energy, balanced and whole. Their love-making is timeless, playful, expansive, and ecstatic. Each small movement has become the most exquisite pleasure. Orgasm has become an ongoing all-over body phenomenon; every cell vibrates to the music of love. They may choose to move into genital release, or not. The goal has completely disappeared. Being one, they are now at peace with whatever the moment brings. From this height, the letting go into a third valley is like a feather, floating softly down in a ray of sunlight. Who can say what is up or what is down? Peak and valley, Yin and Yang, have merged into a single whole.

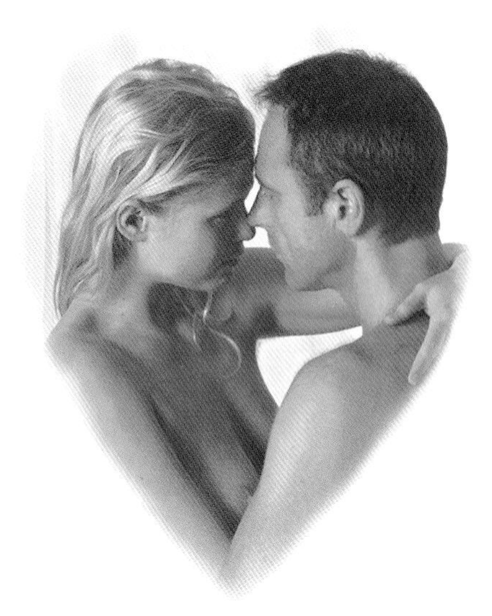

Honoring the feminine and masculine

The scenario described on page 117 gives you an idea of how you can play with the naturally occurring waves of Yin and Yang as they arise during lovemaking. You can continue with this type of lovemaking for as long as you like. It may or may not come into orgasm. You may finish the love session after one peak and one valley, after two peaks and one valley, or after three peaks and three valleys, whatever feels right in the moment.

This style of lovemaking honors both the feminine and the masculine, and so is deeply fulfilling for both. When the Yang is uppermost, it fulfils the needs of the man's body and psyche. It also gives deep nourishment to the woman, as if she is eating the food her soul longs for. This is because the male energy is vital nourishment for her, awakening her own inner male aspect which she cannot feel whole without.

When the Yin is uppermost, the woman can let go deeply into an expansion of her feminine nature. Here her femininity becomes ever more succulent, vast, and mysterious. The man, because he is resting, is then able to absorb the very essence of the feminine, which nurtures a deep longing of his soul. He discovers that he can trust the natural ways energy functions, and thus is relieved from performance anxiety. By letting go deeply into Yin, he allows new sources of Yang energy to spring up as never before.

Naturally, when a couple is able to honor both feminine and masculine aspects during lovemaking, they become deeply intimate. Because both have experienced their longings being met, they feel an overflowing love and gratitude toward each other. Each love session becomes an exploration into the unknown, just listening and being alert to what is naturally occurring in the alchemy of their union.

When the couple experience three cycles of Yin and Yang in a lovemaking session, there is no loss of energy for the man, even if he ejaculates. This is because by the third peak they have created an equal circle of energy, where both man and woman are recharging each other continually. This state is called "The Great Life Renewing Union".

To attain it, you simply need the courage to be very honest with what is happening with your energy in the moment. Drop all performance-oriented moves. Be simple, childlike, playful, and total. If you are lukewarm in your lovemaking, you will move neither to a peak nor to a valley. Totality is vital.

Fear can sometimes prevent couples from experiencing this type of union. The valley represents death as well as renewal; total let go and relaxation is a kind of small death. It is a letting go of your separate identity and experiencing a merging with the source, which holds both great longing and great fear. The fear is there simply because you are letting go of control, and something bigger than you is taking over. If you allow this process you will discover an ego-less state of being, rather like a small infant experiences life. However, as an infant experiencing this state you were unconscious. When you experience it as an adult you are conscious and therefore it becomes a spiritually transforming experience. Mystics call it a second birth. Lovemaking is one of the best ways to dissolve all boundaries and enter into an oceanic oneness, not only with your lover but with the whole universe.

Vernon, a finance manager, is 59 years old, and Valerie, a holistic healing therapist, is 58. They have been married for 17 years. They were introduced to the method of including Yin and Yang during lovemaking in a Tantra group.

Valerie: Making love in Yin and Yang reminded us of when we were first together. We used to go on for hours, and make love more than once. I now realize that this was so fulfilling because it naturally allowed space for the quality of Yin. Practicing lovemaking with three peaks and three valleys took us back in time, as if we were new lovers again. I experienced the same feeling of satisfaction again.

Vernon: We went to the peak, but not over the top into ejaculation. We just floated gently down from there into the valley. The next time we went to an even higher peak. This building up to the peak three times rejuvenates the libido. It was a marvellous feeling.

Valerie: This method is especially good for older people whose libido may be flagging.

Vernon: I have had erection problems, but this time, my erection was much harder and bigger. To move into three peaks and three valleys was simply tremendous.

Valerie: It relieves performance anxiety for both of us. Very often, I have been in a hurry to catch up during sex, trying to reach orgasm before or at the same time as Vernon. Giving space to both Yin and Yang removes that kind of pressure completely.

Vernon: This style of lovemaking gives space for both of us. We are discovering a tremendous sense of closeness, especially coming into the Yin valley. Just lying together, sinking deeper and deeper into intimacy, brings a whole new possibility into our relationship.

chapter 15

foreplay and after-play

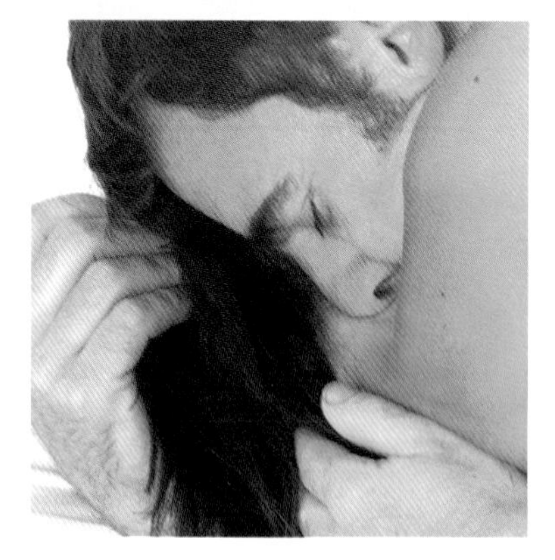

"Whisper those sweet words into my ear
Make my mind smoulder
Come over here
Give me some romance
Just this one time"
Francis Bacon

Sex merits an ambience that raises it high on a pedestal of human attention. After all, it is the sacred ground from which the human race emerges. It also provides a possibility of deep physical, emotional, psychological, and spiritual nourishment. Sex puts a spring in the step, roses in the cheeks, and a song in the heart.

As an act that may bring new life into the world, sex is worthy of some quality attention. You can approach it like fast food, to satisfy your hunger quickly. But if only fast food were available and you could never enjoy a leisurely and elegant dinner with all its rituals, life would be a great deal poorer. This comparison of food with sex is natural, since we have an appetite for both, and both involve pleasure from the senses.

If you go to an elegant restaurant for dinner, you probably take time to prepare, bathing and dressing carefully. At the restaurant, before the main meal arrives you enjoy the apéritif and hors d'oeuvres. The restaurant's atmosphere contributes to your pleasure: the white starched tablecloth, the candles, and perhaps a pianist playing beautiful music.

Yet people rarely give this kind of elegant, ritualistic, and relaxed attention to the sex act. Ancient texts tell us that our ancestors in India, China, Japan, and the Middle East all placed a great deal of importance on creating a special atmosphere for the sex act. You may think that you do not have time for this, but people pursue and put energy into those aspects of life they think are important. If fulfilling sex is at the bottom of your list of things to do during the day, then certainly it will not be a nourishing experience.

People generally have no problem making appointments for business meetings, the hairdresser, or shopping. However, you rarely find a couple scheduling a date for quality lovemaking time together. Make it a priority to get time for yourselves; pay a babysitter if you need to. Creating a beautiful nurturing space together like this will revolutionize your relationship.

Foreplay

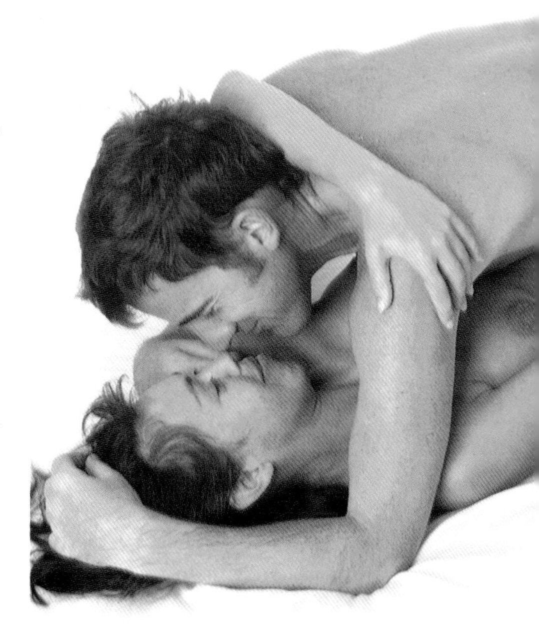

Since women have begun to own their right to enjoy orgasm, a lot of attention has been given to foreplay. This is considered to be the "warm up" before the act of penetration and orgasm. It carries within it an attitude that it is something "added on" to the sex act. This subtle judgement needs to change, otherwise women will continue to feel guilty for something that is to them an essential aspect of a love session. Because a woman's access to pleasure is triggered through whole-body arousal, particularly of her breasts and belly, the sex act will feel one-sided if the man dives straight for the Yoni, thinking only of "the goal" and what gives him pleasure.

Many men would like to please their partner, and erroneously think this will be achieved if they touch her clitoris for a few moments before penetration. Many women simply close up like a clam with this type of goal-oriented touch. When the sex act is one-sided, when male and female energies are not recharging each other in an equal flow of Yin and Yang, it is not satisfying for either partner. There will always be a nagging feeling that something is not right.

Rather than complaining, a woman can affirm her needs clearly. If she is not sure what her needs are, she can ask her man to embark on "trial experiments". It is natural for the woman to be the initiator in Tantra exploration. A woman needs first and foremost to feel loved, cherished, and honored. Her "emotional being" needs to feel connected to her partner, and then her Yoni will open like a flower in the sun. Many women say that they have never felt more sensually alive than when they were teenagers, just playing around, kissing and caressing for hours with a boyfriend, with no goal of penetrative sex. After using the caressing meditation (see page 157) with a partner, many women have told us that it fulfilled something they have been craving for as long as they can remember.

This quality of sensuality needs to be incorporated as an integral part of the sex act, not considered as extra to it. Research by sex therapists has shown that 20 minutes of love play before penetration is the normal amount of time needed for a woman to move into whole-body arousal.

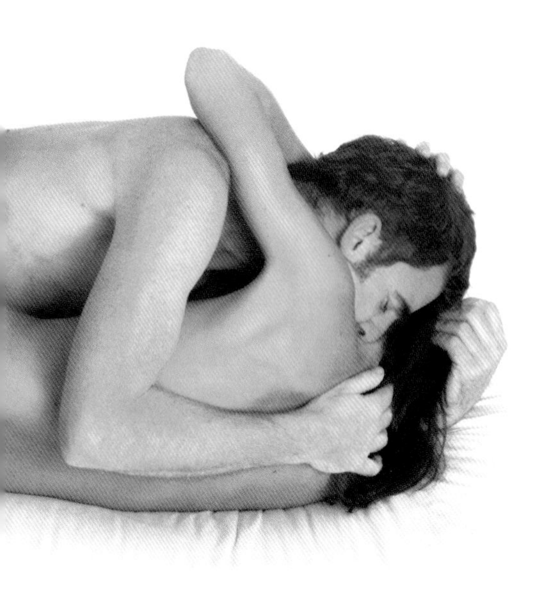

Bring sensitivity and intelligence to each love session, and you will see the beginning and the ending form a circle of loving that goes beyond time. In this way ecstatic sex becomes beginningless and endless – your whole life is drawn into a circle of loving.

Men also have a need to be accepted, loved, and honored for who they are before and during penetrative sex. A wise woman will affirm through words her love and appreciation for her man. Since a man's main positive pole is at the genitals, he needs to be honored there, so that he can really celebrate himself. He will then relax and his heart will open as never before. Once you have honored his Lingam through loving touch, spread this sensual energy all over his body, with kisses, caresses, or massage. After such attention, he may find it easier to continue in lovemaking for a longer time.

A women's sexuality is more connected to the kinaesthetic sense, so the right touch, caresses, and emotional connection are important to her. A man's sexuality is more connected to his visual sense, so sexual images or pornography are attractive to him. "Yoni gazing", one of the meditations used in Tantra, refines this natural inclination and opens access to "inner vision". With inner vision the man becomes aware of deeper energetic layers within his and his partner's body. In this sacred act of meditation, the woman opens her legs and the man sits silently and respectfully, meditating for 20 minutes on the Yoni.

Relaxation, acceptance, and love are keys for entry into sex. At first it may feel strange to enter sexual play in a relaxed manner, without a performance-oriented goal. The man may lose his erection, but it is very natural during foreplay to lose erection, have it come back, and lose it again. Because men tend to think they have to keep an erection all the time, they often find it difficult to relax in foreplay. Don't worry. Whatever needs to happen will happen and you can trust the changing rhythms. You both need to ask yourselves, "Am I connected to myself?" and "Am I connected to my lover?" If that connectedness is not there, love him or her more, and find a way to express that, through your touch, your eyes, your laughter and tears, or through nourishing words.

Ecstasy is born from the meeting of two very alive opposite polarities. Nurture the male and female positive poles and great electricity occurs. The Tantric meditations in this book help lovers to unify their energies and deepen their connection, unveiling the incredible potential contained in sexual union, so that fulfilment is attained.

After-play

When the sex act seems complete, it is not yet over. Take time to express your gratitude to each other in "after-play". This may involve caressing each other all over while murmuring your appreciation, or a romantic dance together. Let after-play be a life-affirming celebration of love.

It may be wonderful to sleep after sex. When sex has been an exquisite fulfilment for both partners, there is a delicious letting go into a restful state together, merged as one in deep embrace. But the cliché of the man who turns over and starts snoring right after his ejaculation, leaving the woman to cry silently into her pillow, is unfortunately a fact for many couples. This happens when the bio-electric circuit between male and female polarities has not been established, so the sex act is little more than the man experiencing genital release inside the woman. He will naturally feel quite drained after such an experience and just want to sleep. The woman may also have experienced genital release, but their positive and receptive poles have not connected enough for them to recharge each other. The woman arrives at a plateau of sexual desire, which continues to vibrate for around 20 minutes after the man has rolled over and gone to sleep. Naturally, the woman will feel extremely frustrated by this. She may relieve herself through self-pleasuring, or she may cry or feel angry, worrying that something is wrong with her or her partner.

If as a couple, you find yourselves in separate worlds after sex, try "Exploring the peaks and valleys of love" (see page 117). This will create a bio-electric current between you that brings wholeness during sex, and a sense of balance at its completion.

You may think that nature has played an unfair trick. Men are eager for a quick consummation of sex and one orgasm, followed by a desire to sleep, while women enjoy a slow build-up and several orgasms, followed by increased energy. But this seeming contradiction gives the spice to sex; a couple has to learn how to mix the spices so that the meal is delicious rather than inedible. To do this you need to work with the ingredients nature has given you, rather than complaining about them; to accept what is and use it creatively.

enhance your love session

♡ Decorate your love chamber to enhance your love session. This may mean using a special bedcover or sheet, candles, scented lamps or incense, plants or flowers, soft lighting, and perhaps music. Clean the space and prepare it before your date.

♡ Shower or bathe to prepare your body.

♡ Think of sex as a sacred celebration of love. Take time to enjoy the beauty of your lover, and each aspect of the sex act. Whisper your appreciation of each other. Caress every part of each other's bodies. Look into each other's eyes for long periods. Hold each other for long moments, absorbing the scents of hidden and secret parts of the body. Kiss, lick, and nibble each other all over.

♡ Make sounds of delirious pleasure. Delight in the miracle of love. Let your emotions flow as you express wild abandon with your lover. Sex is a flowing phenomenon. What happens before penetration is as much part of it as what happens in the middle or at the conclusion. Experience each aspect of the symphony of sexual love in its fullness.

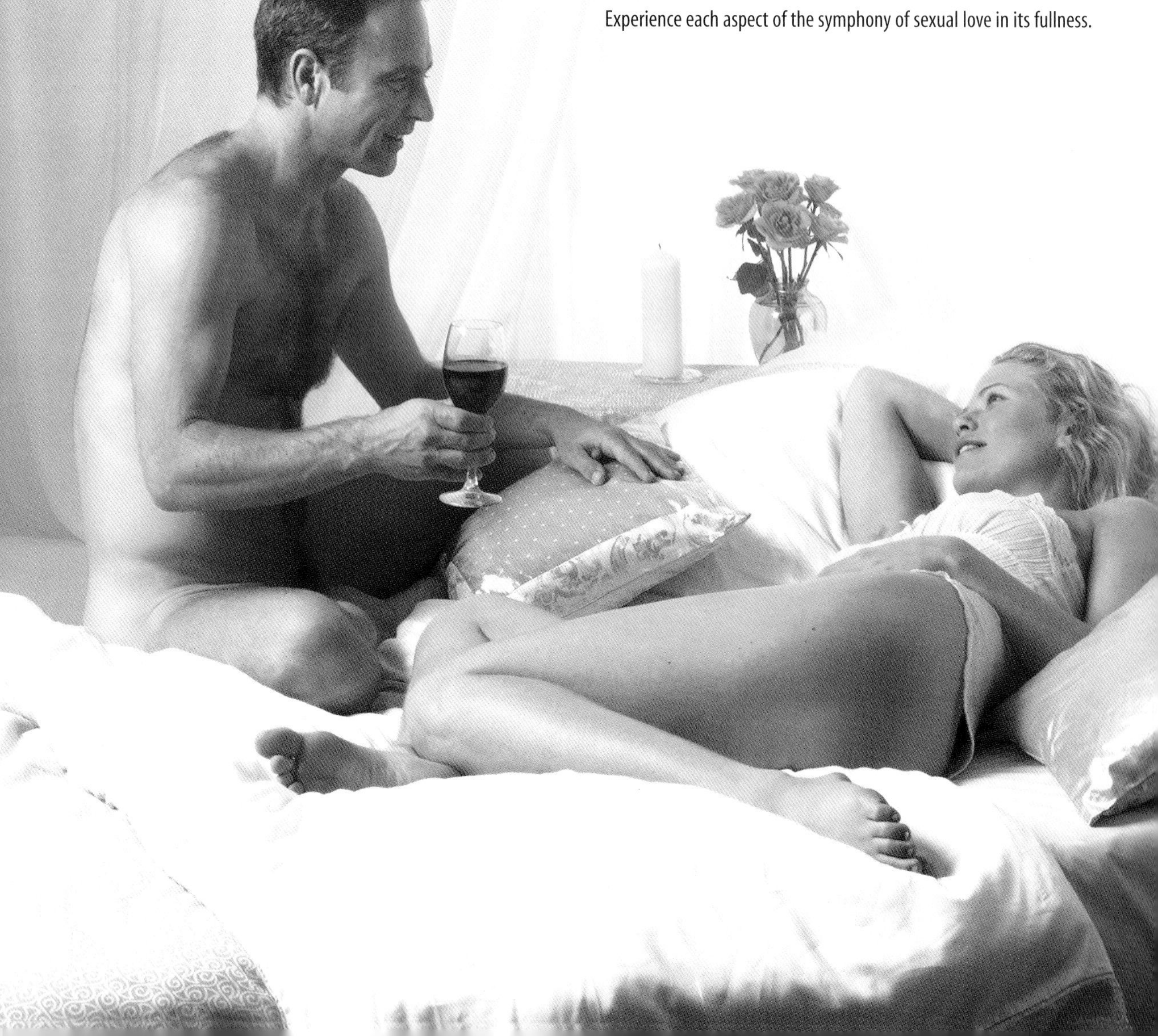

intelligent refinement of sex

♡ Clearly 11 o'clock at night is not always the best time to have sex. It is wise to be rested before sex.

♡ If the woman loves to have a few orgasms, and is often frustrated that the game is over just as she is getting started, the couple needs to spend more time in foreplay. During foreplay, do not just focus on the woman's pleasure as a tedious routine before penetration. Both man and woman need equal space to savor the delights of a whole-body awakening of pleasure. This will help you to synchronize so that you recharge each other moment by moment during sex.

♡ Aiming for one simultaneous orgasm may put strain and stress on both of you. Let yourself be more playful. Drop the goal and just follow your natural sexual urges. A woman may like to have a few orgasms before penetration, just to be really open and ready for her man. This is usually a better approach than trying to satisfy her after the man has already had an orgasm. The more time pressure there is on a woman to orgasm, the less likely she will be able to do so.

♡ It may not be best for both partners to orgasm each time you make love. The man may wish to conserve his energy or the woman may not be at a time in her cycle where she feels the need to orgasm.

♡ It is important to have sharing times outside of sex, to talk about how things are going and what might need some loving consideration, giving equal time for both partners to be heard. It is also important not to keep any secrets from each other, as secrets will slowly erode intimacy. To be really in tune during sex means you both need to be wide open, exposed to each other, with nothing to hide.

♡ The more love and acceptance there is between partners, the easier sex will be. Find more ways of expressing your love to your partner, and you will see your relationship flowering.

♡ After-play is an overflowing of love and appreciation after a deeply nurturing and fulfilling sexual union. If you are overflowing with joy, you may want to demonstrate this with some joyful act, like serving breakfast in bed, or washing your partner all over in the shower, or covering your lover from head to toe with kisses.

♡ If your sexual union has gone very deep, merging you not only physically but also on a soul level, the best expression of love may be to meditate silently next to each other, savoring the sweetness and feeling gratefulness lifting you higher. Meditation after lovemaking may bring you into a vastness of love, which seems to have no beginning and no ending. You can bathe in this space for some time and then bow down to each other in recognition of your divine natures.

♡ If gratitude and overflowing energy are not present at the end of a sexual meeting, you need to bring more awareness to the beginning and the middle of your sexual union. Something is not in balance. As your approach to sex becomes more refined, after-play will become an effortless expression of your joy and fulfilment.

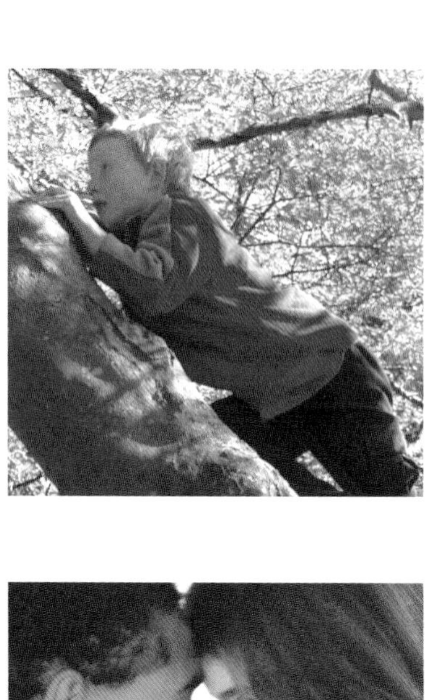
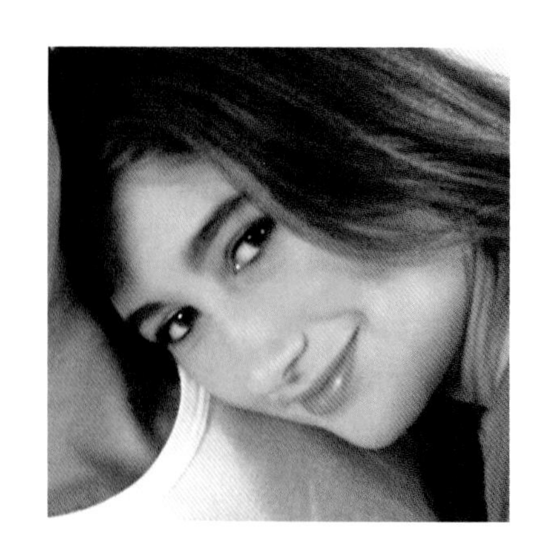
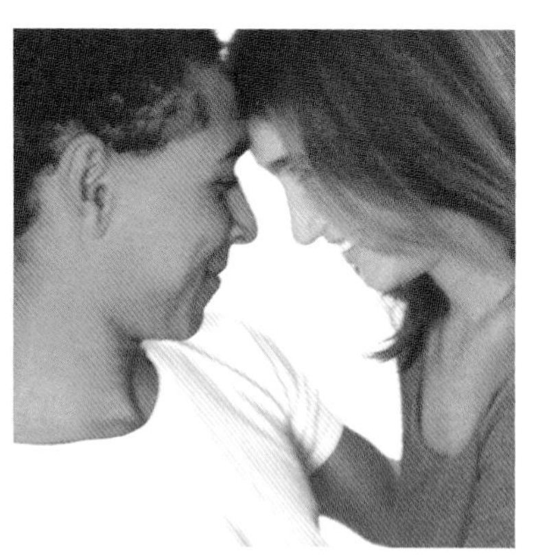
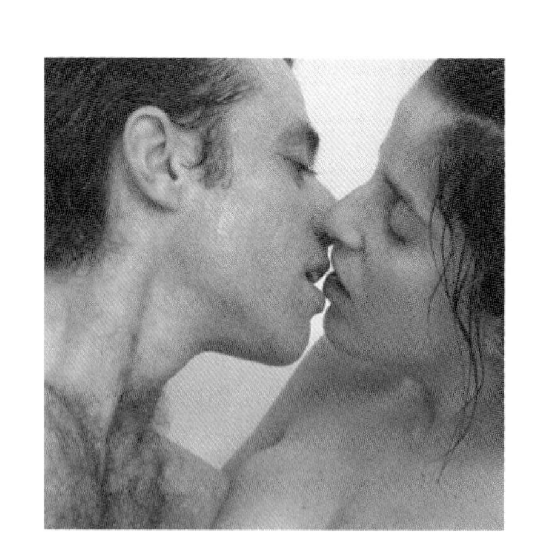
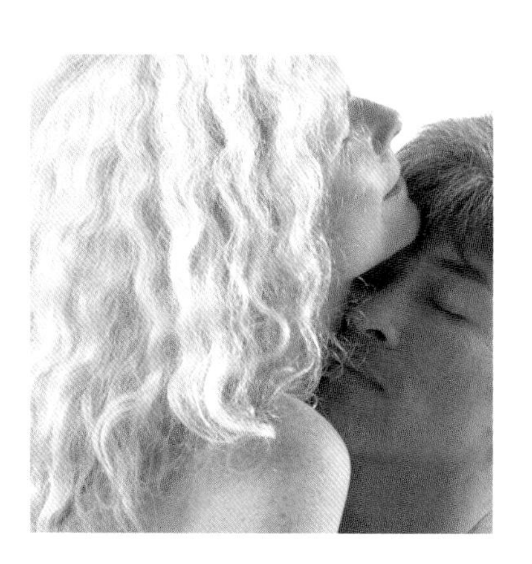
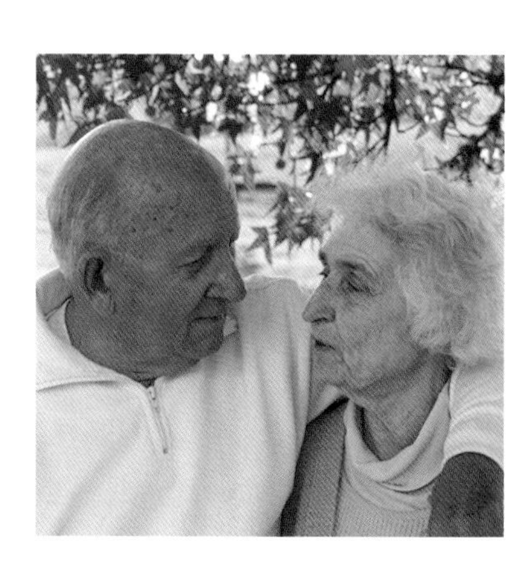

part 5

the ages of love

In life we move through seven-year cycles, each ending with a transmutation into a new state of being. In much the same way as a butterfly emerges from a cocoon, we evolve to new levels of exploration and freedom, in body, emotion, psychological expression, and soul development. These phases play an important role in our unfolding as fulfilled sexual human beings.

If you can tune into the changes that would like to occur at these moments of transition, and allow yourself to open up new avenues of expression, you will know continuous evolution toward light, bliss, and freedom. Each previous stage of development will be absorbed as fuel for the next in an ever-expanding spiral dance of learning and transformation. If you hinder the transition, then you prevent the river of life flowing, causing stagnation of growth and evolution.

When the flow of life is encouraged, the older we become, the more we have access to understanding and plenitude. We can learn to integrate all experience into a rich multidimensional expression – a rainbow of love, creativity, and wisdom.

chapter 16

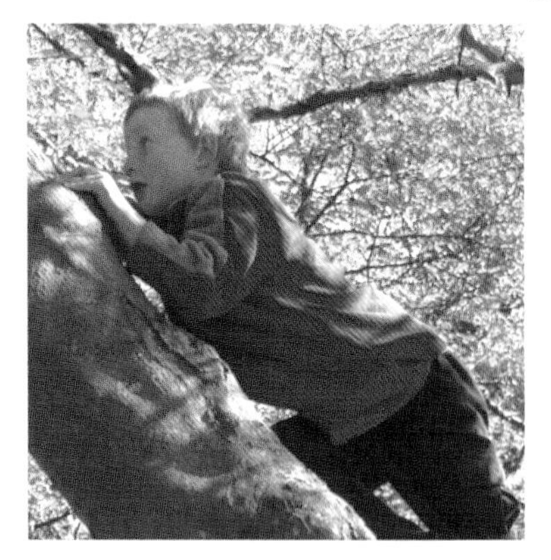

sensuality of the child

"Tenderness is learned by receiving it – from babyhood onwards. The real lessons about relationships are learned by age three."
From *Raising Boys*, Steve Biddulph

Childhood can be divided into two seven-year cycles, from birth to seven, and from seven to 14 years. Within both of these seven-year cycles, there is no sexual connotation in any of the child's actions. It is not part of children's nature, because they are not yet producing the hormones that make sexual feelings a reality. However, they have sensual and pleasurable feelings, even orgasmic rushes of energy through the genitals and the whole body. A child passionately seeks body contact, sensual experiences, and ways of giving and receiving love as he or she moves nearer to the time of independence. Children are programmed to explore through imitation the adult behaviour they witness. Later on, even if they do not wish to continue exhibiting this behavior, and fight against it, they will find themselves repeating it.

The more that children can be encouraged to develop their own resourceful, creative endeavours, the more their intelligence will expand. Sitting too long in front of the TV dampens children's ability to think for themselves, and may warp their understanding of reality. Learning is a process of drawing out the innate and unique potential a child carries inside. The more space a child has just to be with his or her own inner resources, particularly in nature, the more creativity will spring forth.

The three principal qualities of support for a growing child are love, sincerity, and silent contemplation. These qualities nurture gratefulness toward life and a desire to enhance life through creative expression. Love between people, and reverence and care for nature and the environment are important factors in a child's learning. Sincerity and honesty in adults' speech and action will nurture sincerity in the child. If the family meditates together, spending some time in silence each day, this will be greatly beneficial to the child's development. You can use Silent Meditation (see chapter 24) or the Children's meditation technique on page 132, letting the child meditate for as long as he or she wishes.

A firm foundation in love, sincerity, and meditation will encourage the hormonal changes of puberty, when they come, to seek expression along these pathways that were established in childhood. The adult who will emerge from such a foundation will be both loving and wise.

From birth to seven years

The first seven years could be described as the self-pleasuring phase, because the child is concerned primarily with him- or herself as the center of the universe. Everything revolves around his or her individual needs being met. Children in this phase are in a way helpless, and yet they also find very inventive ways of amusing themselves. The whole world is simply there as a playground in which to learn and absorb continuously. It is a very vulnerable time, when any input from adults will be absorbed either for good or ill. Because children feel themselves to be the central character in life, they will also blame themselves if anything goes wrong. For example, if the parents are fighting and unhappy, the child will feel he or she is to blame.

In this period children very naturally touch and explore their own bodies, finding pleasure in stroking the skin, or bathing, or the feel of the sun and wind. The young child is totally alive with each sensory experience, whether this involves seeing, hearing, smelling, tasting, or feeling. The child also loves to touch his or her own genitals, discovering this area as a place full of mystery and pleasure, which brings aliveness all over the body as well as deep nurturing and relaxation. This innocent pleasure, which benefits the child's growth hormones, should not be discouraged. It is natural for a baby boy to have erections, as he has quite a lot of testosterone in his body at this time. If he is uncircumcised, it is natural for him to feel the need to massage his foreskin, in this way gradually freeing its mobility.

The child has no judgement about good or bad, higher or lower, animal or divine. It is a time of original innocence and wonder. Pleasure exists in all the small discoveries of life, such as learning to eat, to dress, to sing, or to paint. Each activity overflows with innocent sensuality. The child has the ability to live completely in the moment. When the child laughs, he or she

"In the 1960s, anthropologist James Prescott carried out a very large scale study of child rearing and violence across different societies. He found that those societies which gave less touching and affection to young children, had by far the most violence amongst adults. It's clear that the more tender and warm are the lives of children, the safer and more loving they will be as adults."

From *Raising Boys*, by Steve Biddulph

becomes just laughter, expressed through the entire body. A child is a reminder to the adult of how to live in the moment, one of the greatest keys to a fulfilling life.

The more love children receive during their first seven years, the more they will overflow with love when they reach adulthood. Before a fountain can overflow, it has to be filled with water. Before a child can grow up to be a loving adult, he or she needs to learn what love is through receiving it. This love needs to be given unconditionally. The whole game of, "If you are good, I will love you", is destructive. Love means cuddling, reading stories together, walking in nature, kneeling down to the child's level and making eye contact when you want to impart something, playing together and listening deeply when there is something the child would like to express.

From seven to fourteen years

In the second seven-year cycle the child becomes curious about the surrounding world and will develop friendships with other children. It is a phase of same-sex relating, which is a non-threatening way to experience how it is to become intimate with other human beings. The child sees him or herself in the mirror of another child and develops intimate ways of playing, touching, and relating. Children may develop innocent same sex or opposite sex love affairs, in which they copy or play-act what they have seen between adults. Playing doctors, or mums and dads, gives them a chance to explore bodies and relationships. Some children have been traumatized for life by parents screaming at them when they were innocently playing together in the nude.

"Listen to what kids want. Don't lose it with them."

Rob, age 12

Normal schooling relies mainly on the visual and auditory senses, which suits a lot of people. But some teachers have found that children who are apparently slow to learn suddenly excel when they are guided to learn through physical games or experiences, thus enabling them to absorb the teaching kinaesthetically. Ideally education should use all the senses, to allow children to learn in their own unique style.

During this phase, the sense of "I" as an individual develops. The desire to learn more of life is unquenchable, and yet children need very secure boundaries – to feel utterly safe and secure in the daily routine, with emotional support and love in a protected learning environment. You can see this in the animal kingdom: young puppies or cubs are adventurous and bold, playing at being fierce hunters, but they are never far from their mother's watchful eye and protection.

Sexual abuse

Sexual exploitation of children and child pornography appear to be escalating in western society. Parents need to monitor how, when, and where the protective boundaries are opened as the child grows toward independence. However, some parents have become afraid to touch their children at all for fear of traumatizing them sexually. This is misguided, since affection, intimacy, and physical contact are essential for the nurturing of the child.

Listen carefully to what your child would like to say and teach your child that their own and everyone else's genitals are private parts. If anyone asks them to show or do things with their private parts, then the child must shout "NO!" and ask an adult for help as soon as possible, even if they have been told to keep the activity a secret. Let them know clearly that they are allowed to say no to another person, no matter who that person may be.

As healers and in Tantra groups, we have worked with many adults who were sexually abused as children. Sexual abuse destroys the child's ability to grow and develop naturally. It is never under any circumstances beneficial to either the child or the adult involved. It harms the child so deeply that he or she will need years of therapy and healing on every level of body, mind, and soul to recover from it. A child who is repeatedly abused may become programmed to repeat the same behaviour as an adult, unless they receive adequate therapy to release the trauma. At the very least, their sexual response will be damaged.

Many abusing adults were themselves abused as children. This trauma may have been buried in the subconscious and the adult may be surprised and even shocked by his or her own behavior. Any adult who is uneasy with their sexuality should consult a therapist who is competent to help with sexual issues. The desire for perverted sex always stems from unhealthy attitudes and/or experiences during childhood.

Helena Vistara is an Education Consultant, Counsellor and Family Therapist and founder of Creative Parenting, which supports families in natural and empowering ways of living, loving, and learning. She defines sexual abuse as "any sexually stimulating activity that exploits a child's natural open-hearted disposition, or their desire for physical contact and sensual experience".

Sexual abuse includes:

1) Looking at the child with sexual intent.

2) Touching a child with sexual desire and innuendo.

3) Asking or encouraging a child to touch his or her own genitals sexually or to engage in sexually provocative activities.

4) Touching a child's genitals sexually.

5) A request by an adult for the child to touch the adult's genitals.

6) Engaging in sex with the child, either anal, vaginal or oral.

7) Asking or encouraging a child to watch others engaged in masturbation or sexual activity, including home movies, TV, or video.

tips for a healthy sexual environment

♡ Children benefit from their parents demonstrating affection: hugging and kissing, tenderness and intimacy, flirting and laughing together. They also benefit from a relaxed attitude around nudity.

♡ Answer children's questions about sex at the correct level for their development and understanding. It is a good idea to pause before answering a child's question. In the pause they may answer it themselves, if they simply wanted to know that someone was listening. The listening pause also gives them time to make more clear what information they are seeking. Do not give too much detail at one time; if the child wishes to know more they will ask.

♡ When a child shows signs of physical development leading toward puberty, around age 9 or 10, explain the full facts of sexual life to them if they haven't yet asked about it, even if they have already learned about it in school. You may like to use a step-by-step approach, giving the child time to ponder over what they have learned and ask any questions after each step. Parents can share some of their own personal experiences: how they learned about sex and what is important to them, particularly the pleasure and fulfilment that comes with intimate love.

♡ Explain to both boys and girls how their bodies will develop in puberty, and about menstruation, so that they are informed about themselves and the opposite sex. Going with her mother to purchase her first bra is a big event in a girl's life, an affirmation that she is growing into womanhood. A boy may need to buy underwear suitable for protecting his testicles during sports.

♡ As children reach puberty, they need privacy in order to feel free to explore their new physical developments. Sexual openness, warmth, and honesty from the very beginning will help each important transition to happen in a celebrative way.

children's meditation

This technique was developed by Osho, a contemporary Tantra master.

♡ **Step 1** Ten minutes' gibberish. Make nonsense sounds in any language you don't know, while roaming around, moving your body freely.

♡ **Step 2** Ten minutes' belly laughter, with eyes open or closed. (There does not need to be any reason for the laughter. It is an exercise in learning to laugh freely, not needing an outside cause to provoke it.)

♡ **Step 3** Ten minutes' silence, either sitting or lying down, with eyes closed. Become aware of your body and thoughts as a detached witness, without any judgement.

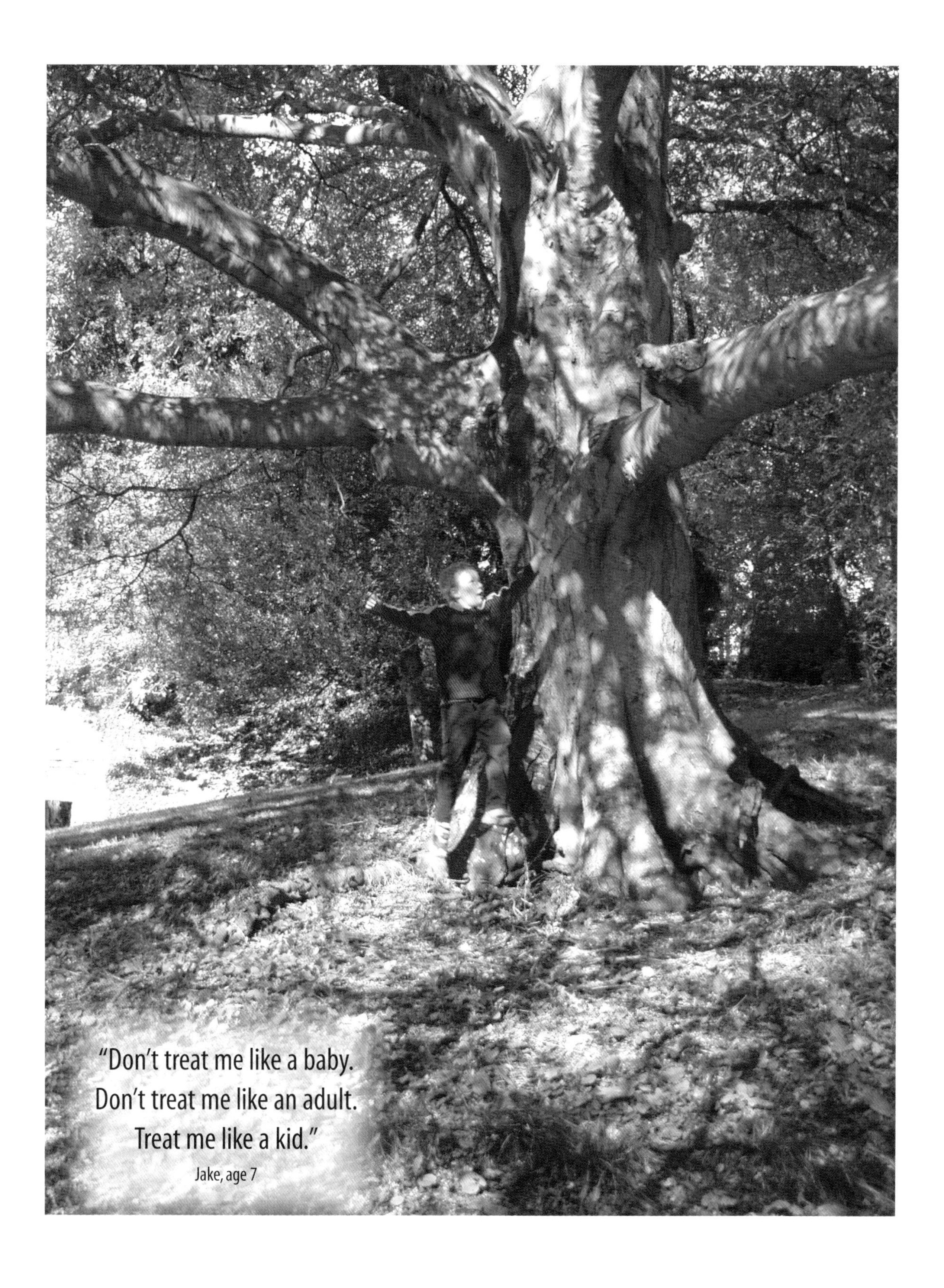
"Don't treat me like a baby.
Don't treat me like an adult.
Treat me like a kid."
Jake, age 7

chapter 17

sexual awakening at adolescence

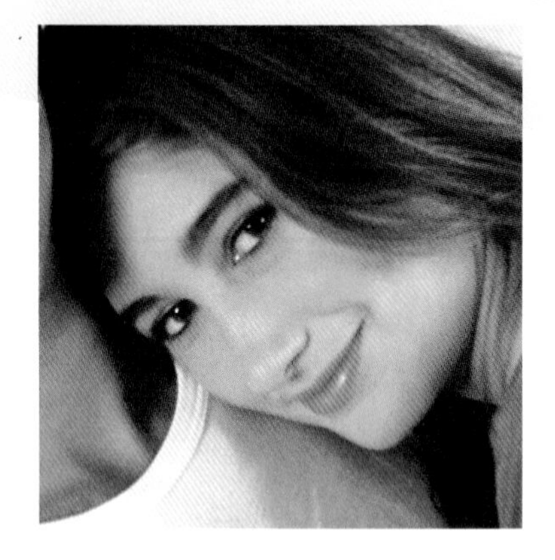

"I had three friends
One asked me to sleep on the mat
One asked me to sleep on the ground
One asked me to sleep on his breast
I decided to sleep on his breast
I saw myself carried on a river
I saw the king of the river
And the king of the sun"
Traditional Nigerian song

The dawning of adolescence brings with it a revolution. Who the child is in their innermost psyche will suddenly burst forth, like a sprout that now reveals the type of plant it will become. Hormonal changes – secretion of estrogens and progesterone in girls and testosterone in boys – cause physical transformation. Like a young sapling, the child may suddenly shoot upward at a phenomenal rate of growth. The voice will gain a deeper timbre. In girls the hips and breasts will swell. Pubic and underarm hair will develop. The odor of hormonal readiness for sensual exploration will begin attracting the opposite sex.

It is a time for a testing your own power and boundaries. The intense desire to discover your own individual truth and express it is overwhelming. The adolescent will either respect the parents and develop lifelong bonding as friends, or will rebel against parental hypocrisy. How he or she responds depends on how honest, loving, and wise the parents were through his or her childhood – they are weighed in the scale of their past actions.

"When a child is young they need strong roots. When they become a teenager, they need roots and wings. A parent has to be ready to let go, and at the same time, needs to provide a safe and nurturing rooted space for them to come back to. You really need to touch and cuddle a young teenager a lot, otherwise they may go into sex before they're ready, just to get some emotional security through touch."

Charaka, holistic health therapist, teacher, and mother

During these years sexual desire begins to bubble up. Many people have a fear of allowing their young ones to indulge in free sexual experimentation. However, nature demands that the young explore sex as freely as possible. They are searching for the highest peaks that the drug of their own hormones can bring, and this means experimentation without attachment. If they have had a solid foundation of love and sincerity in childhood and are educated about the facts of life, they can be trusted to become a pioneer in sex, though they need to feel that an adult is there for guidance when they need it. If teenagers do not have this freedom they may be incapable of intimacy as adults because they remain "stuck" in adolescence. However, adolescents should not be pushed into sex before they are ready.

Each teenager has their own rate of growth and development. When the girl has her first period, it does not mean she is ready for a sexual relationship. She may need a slow entry into puberty, learning to kiss, caress, and generally experience the thrill of pleasure, getting used to sensing her provocative power. A boy may need a phase of male bonding during puberty, in order to become fully grounded in his manhood. For both, the onset of puberty demands strong same-sex role models, through which they will become empowered on their journey into maturity.

Teenagers are extremely vulnerable and insecure and may try to hide this behind a veneer of bravado. Their bodies are changing rapidly, they have peer pressure to excel as a sexually desirable person, and also they are expected to show signs of adult responsibility by getting good grades, planning a career, finding work, and so on. They need to know that their parents respect their intelligence, and find them good company and nice to have around. Sometimes it is good for parents to seek their advice, with genuine curiosity.

Steve Biddulph, in his inspiring book *Raising boys*, recounts a wonderful initiation ceremony for young men. The boys, together with their fathers or an older male friend, go on a camping trip together. During the weekend, they spend an evening around the fire, each adult telling stories and lessons he has learned from his own life, as well as affirming the positive qualities of the boy and expressing his pride in him. The boys, in their turn, speak about their own lives, their values, and their hopes for the future. The fathers then affirm how they can support the boy in his quest.

Rites of passage

With puberty, there needs to be a celebration of an adolescent's new status as young woman rather than little girl, or young man rather than little boy. Aboriginal societies traditionally see a coming of age ceremony as a very important threshold into the world of sexual responsibility.

You can create your own special ceremony for your son or daughter, giving their passage into adulthood the dignity and respect it deserves. A woman we know takes young pubescent girls for a ceremonial swim with dolphins to celebrate their coming of age. Something which is empowering, uplifting, and in celebration of their new role in life will do wonders for the boy/man or girl/woman. Offer them the respect their new step in life deserves and they will in turn respect you.

chapter 18

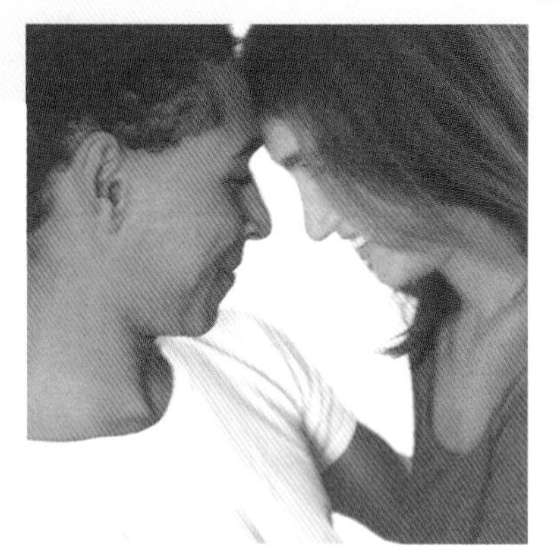

first sexual experiences

"Now she has known first love desires flood her mind. She trembles with delight... She studies her reflection in a jewel, knits her brow, and oh so tenderly touches the blossoming love-bite on her lip."
Vidyapati, India 15th century

In our society, most adolescents learn about sex through TV, videos and magazines. But sexually explicit images, mostly created by men for men, usually represent warped sexual attitudes. They do not demonstrate what a sensual and fulfilling sexuality could look like. The sexual habits you develop at adolescence tend to stay with you and change only through a re-learning process such as Tantra or through teaching from a sexual partner. So it is important to start your sexual life with information that gives a proper direction, toward the ongoing exploration of a more ecstatic love life.

sex tips for girls

♡ Look at the diagrams of the genital anatomy (page 23). Use a mirror to look at your genitals and identify the different parts. Then touch the different areas, so that you can discover what brings the most pleasure to you. Get to know your own body and its potential for pleasure.

♡ Learn to dance in a style that enhances free body movements and sensuality, such as African, belly dance, Five Rhythms, or Mamba.

♡ Learn holistic body massage from a professional. The art of touch is one of the most valuable gifts you can give yourself and others.

♡ If a partner tries to pressure you into sex before you are ready, remember that it is not your responsibility to make him feel better. Your responsibility is toward yourself and your wellbeing. You do not have to have sex; it can be magical just to lie in each other's arms.

♡ When you are ready, take time to create the right ambience for your first sex act. Make sure you understand about birth control and safe sex (see chapter 7). Choose a place that feels special to you, with enough time so that you feel relaxed. Kiss each other, caress, play with each other's bodies. Don't allow penetration until your Yoni is swollen and wet with arousal, on the verge of orgasm. Then the pain of moving through the hymen, if you still have one, will be minimal. (Some girls lose their hymen in ways other than sexual penetration, such as horseback riding or cycling.)

♡ During sex it is natural for both partners to feel very vulnerable and emotional. Let yourself learn, while at the same time trusting your intuition about what feels good and what doesn't. Talk openly to your partner about what you like or don't like.

♡ Love yourself enough to go for what you need. If your partner doesn't know how to turn you on, show him how you like it. Touch and arouse yourself without inhibition, or show him how.

♡ With a lover, if you feel that your heart is expanding and your love is growing, then you are moving in a good direction. If you feel that your heart is shrinking and you are oppressed, then it is a wrong direction. Your heart will guide you toward healthy ways of relating.

♡ Ask an older woman for guidance, but remember that adults are also in an ongoing learning process around sexuality and relating and therefore do not know everything.

♡ Learn as much as you can about your body and its functioning; this knowledge and understanding will serve you well through life.

sex tips for boys

♡ Self-pleasuring is natural and necessary for discovering your own sexuality. Be relaxed, take time, enjoy the slow build-up of energy. Try to make it more of a full-body experience, rather than a localized pleasure in the genitals. Allow your body to move and use sensuous touch, taking you to greater heights of pleasure. Enjoy each moment rather than hankering only for the ejaculation. Refine more and more the art of self-pleasuring by postponing the ejaculation as long as you can. These experiments with yourself will give you the right background for being a sensitive and good lover.

♡ When you are first attracted to a girl, it is very natural to feel awkward and shy. Everyone is shy in this situation, but some people are better at going beyond their fears than others. Approach her and ask if she would like to spend some time with you. If the answer is no, you can feel proud that you had enough courage to express yourself. One day you will meet someone you like who will answer "Yes".

♡ On your first sexual date, don't be afraid to admit that you have no experience in lovemaking. Your partner will relax more and it will be easier and more fun. Don't be afraid to ask a woman to teach you; she may feel honored to initiate you into the joys of lovemaking.

♡ Make sure you know about contraception (see chapter 7). Practice safe sex and wear a condom every time.

♡ A woman will generally only be ready for penetration after at least 20 minutes of foreplay. There is no need to rush to her Yoni to try to turn her on; her whole body needs to become aroused (see chapter 15). Don't worry if you lose your erection. Go on enjoying each other's bodies. When the moment is right, some erection will be there, enough to penetrate. Once inside, the Lingam naturally gets the idea.

♡ When it is time for penetration, go slowly. If you are too active, you will quickly ejaculate, so be easy and sensuous. Go on with caresses and kisses, make soft and sensuous movements, and enjoy this special moment. After around five minutes, there will be a union of body electricity. From then on you can be sensitive to the different waves of energy, sometimes passionate and fiery, sometimes slowing down in a more feminine phase of deep fulfilment (see chapter 14).

♡ Penetration gives a man enough stimulation to bring him to genital orgasm, but for a woman penetration alone is not usually enough. Very few women orgasm without additional stimulation of the clitoris. The best way to discover what your partner likes is by watching her doing it herself. However, your partner may feel too shy to do that, especially the first few times you make love.

♡ To turn an ordinary human love-making moment into a divine experience, keep a feeling of "thank you" in your heart. Then you will elevate this sensuous moment into ecstasy.

♡ Opening the flow of physical energy with free-form dance and massage will contribute a lot to a life of fulfilling sex.

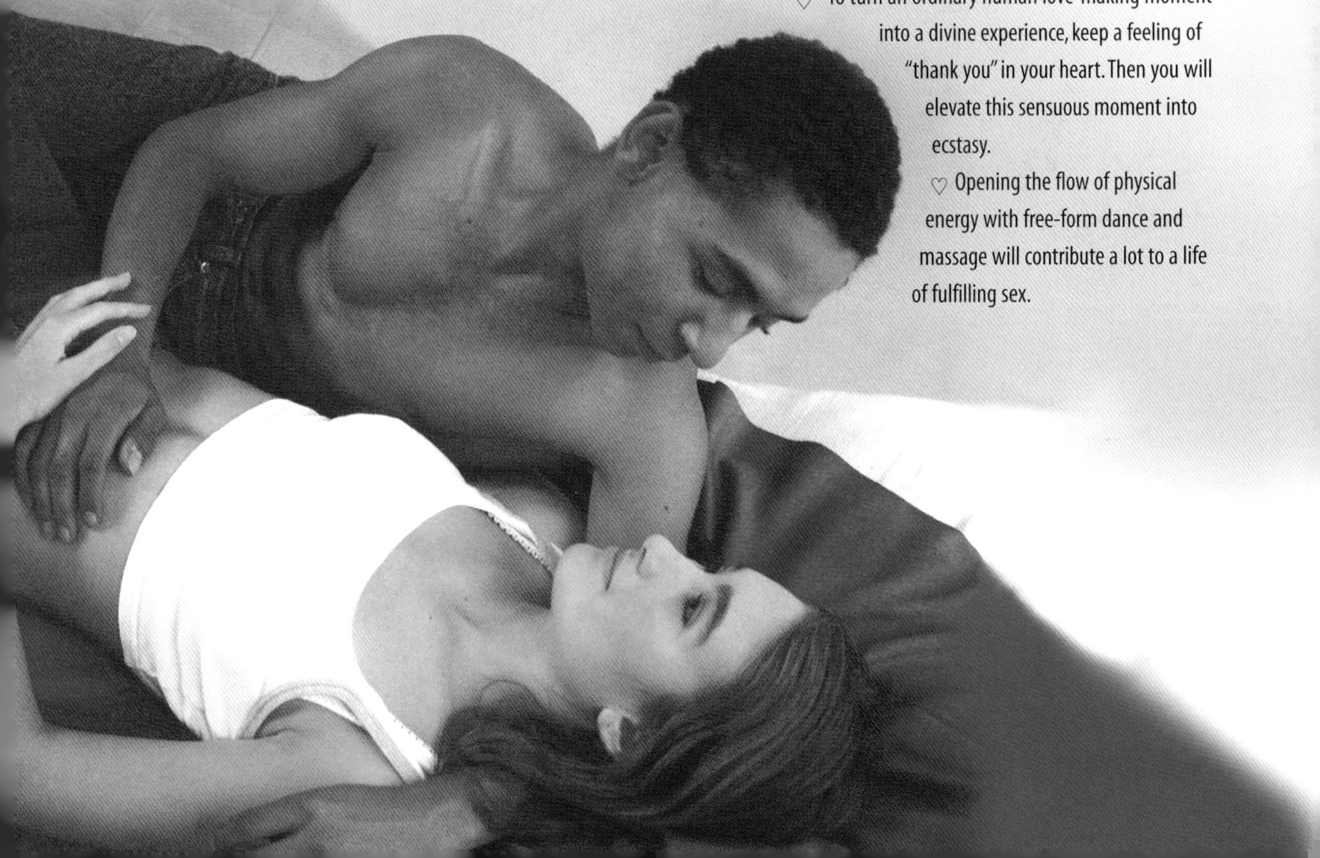

chapter 19

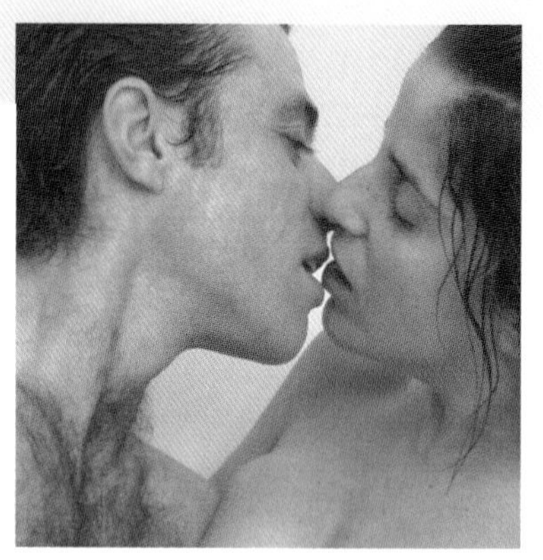

sexuality in young adulthood

"Pillowed on your thighs in a dream garden,
little flower with its perfumed stamen
singing, sipping from the stream of you –
sunset, moonlight - our song continues."
Ikkyu Sojun Zen Master, founder of the "Red Thread" School of Zen, Japan, 15th century

The first phase of adulthood spans three seven-year cycles from 21 to 42. This is a very rich time for sexual exploration and for learning about relationships and how to live in the world.

From 21 to 28

This is when young adults discover the joys and sorrows of intimate relating. They may have one or more deep relationships in which they will be using the other as a mirror to discover their own potential as a lover and as a human being. The young adult is also learning to take on worldly responsibility, which brings its own challenges. It is a time when striving to realize your inner dreams is of paramount importance, whether those dreams are worldly, sexual, or spiritual – or a combination of all three.

In this period it is wise to learn how to care for your body, establishing healthy eating patterns and taking regular exercise, so that as you become older you will remain fit and healthy.

From 28 to 35

This is a time of deep soul-searching and radical transformation. Whatever the person has been living until this time is now questioned. They may feel as though their life is being turned upside down. Relationships may break up, new relationships may form; life direction or career may suddenly change. This happens because nature is giving you a second chance to face yourself and discover your true soul calling. Though it may be difficult, the upheaval will improve your life. If you truly follow the calling of your soul you will become happier and healthier than you have ever been. This phase is about saying "YES" to yourself, whatever form that may take and whatever the cost.

By this time you will have learned quite a lot about sex, love, and relating. You may have burning questions that demand answers. Is true love possible? Should I start a family? Will I ever find the satisfaction I seek sexually? Can sex and spirituality merge? The ship of your life may find turbulent waters as you seek to find answers to these questions. Some people choose to "give up" at this time, finding the challenge of listening to the soul too daunting. If you give up you will pay the price for this decision in the next seven-year cycle when your body begins breaking down – an outward sign of the inner decision to give up.

A woman may be surprised to find her sexuality becoming very succulent in this phase. She may want to have several love affairs or to experiment with different styles of lovemaking and sexual toys. It is a peak time for a woman to express her sensuousness, her juiciness, and her passion – her fullness as a woman seeks expression. If she can embrace this aspect of herself, it will help her to become a wise woman later on, because she will live her full potential without restraint. Just as women generally take longer than men to become fully sexually aroused, they also need time to ease into the fullness of sex, wishing first to become grounded in the dimensions of love and relating.

During this cycle from 28 to 35 years old, practicing Tantra can greatly benefit a couple, as it will help them to merge the fullness of sexual expression with spirituality and love. It will encourage the disparate natures of man and woman to come together in harmony and understanding, teaching invaluable lessons for the continual unfolding of life.

"Making love now is just amazing. We are exploring a whole new landscape. I am in a process of unwinding layers of all kinds of things that were sitting on my natural sexuality. It is a very relaxed process, happening through Tantra.

One of the layers that has dropped is how my sexuality has been dominated by my beliefs. It was scary to drop it, because even though it was a cage it was a known place. But going into the unknown is easier now, because our love has grown deeper, and sweeter. When we make love, the love is already there – we just drop into it."

Divyam (31), Tantra group participant

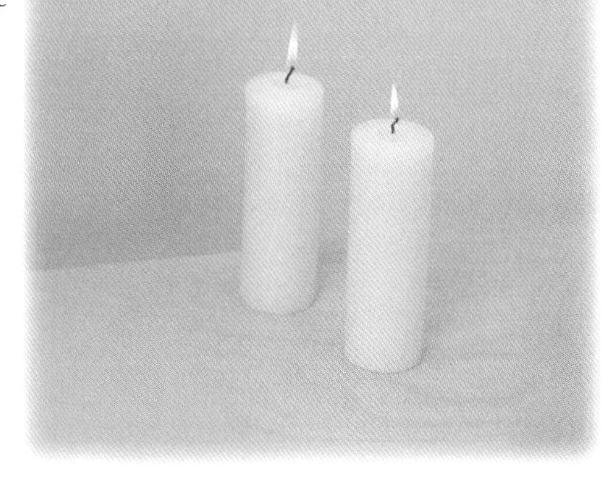

From 35 to 42

Many people have a feeling that after 35 it is all downhill. But this is only true if the person has not listened to their soul calling them to transform in the previous cycle. The fruits of what you have or have not lived in one cycle always show themselves in the seven-year cycle that follows.

If you have missed living what nature intended in one cycle, it is not too late. You can turn your life around and make up for what you have missed in an intense burst of expression. Doing

"I have pleasure beyond what I've ever dreamed. I never knew that you can feel that good and that complete. Being with Divyam now is like coming home. Just lying in her arms is eating the sweetest fruit, beyond Eden. Even just the embrace is orgasm."

Keerti (38), Tantra group participant

this is like removing a dam from the river of your life, allowing the water to flow through again. It is never too late to reclaim the calling of your soul, right up to your last breath.

This period is all about creative expression. All the learning you have absorbed in life so far bursts out into the dimension of sharing and overflowing. You may find yourself teaching, or painting, or creating a garden, or building a house, or starting a family or a business. You begin to master the things that you have been endeavoring to learn throughout your life. For this reason it may be a time of intense fulfilment and happiness, as you surf the waves of your well-deserved achievement. This is the kind of happiness you could never have imagined as you started your journey into young adulthood. You may feel so much more at peace with yourself than you did then. It is truly the cycle of fulfilment.

You may also be discovering an awesome spiritual dimension to sex. At times you may sense that your sexuality can become an experience of deep meditation which transcends all emotional holding patterns. If you are practicing Tantra, you may realize the oneness that is possible with another human being, when all your seven chakras start vibrating as one.

Conversely, if you have not been able to live according to your nature, this may be a time when you risk everything to find happiness. You may start to seek a spiritual master, or to attend personal development groups and classes, or to read every book you can, to discover a way of getting out of the rut you now find yourself in. You may find that your body is showing signs of ill health and begin a radical transformation in your eating and exercise habits. In this case, trust your sense of direction for change. Go toward what uplifts your heart and you will find yourself on the right track.

Men may find a quietening of their sexual urges. They may notice that their erection is not as hard as it used to be, or that they need more time between ejaculations for sexual desire to mount again. In some men this will create anxiety and they will start looking for methods to turn back the clock. Holistic health methods may help to restore health and libido, and learning Tantra will teach you how to expand your life force during sex.

tips for connecting with your lover

In young adulthood, many couples are very busy, trying to organize their lives. When you arrive home at the end of the day full of the stresses of work, it is wise to take time to tune into each other.

♡ Have a meal or a bath together before lovemaking. Don't expect just to come home from your very different experiences in the day and jump straight into great sex. You need a transition phase to unwind together.

♡ For a bath before lovemaking, add essential oils to the water. Rose connects to the heart, while Sandalwood is calming and uplifting, a gentle aphrodisiac that connects sex with spirituality. Check your choice of oils with a qualified practitioner or a book on aromatherapy.

♡ Create a special space. Make a clear agreement that this is your safe time and space to explore together. Turn off the telephone. Clear and prepare your temple of love together.

♡ Show consideration during lovemaking. Check frequently with each other that what you are doing is OK.

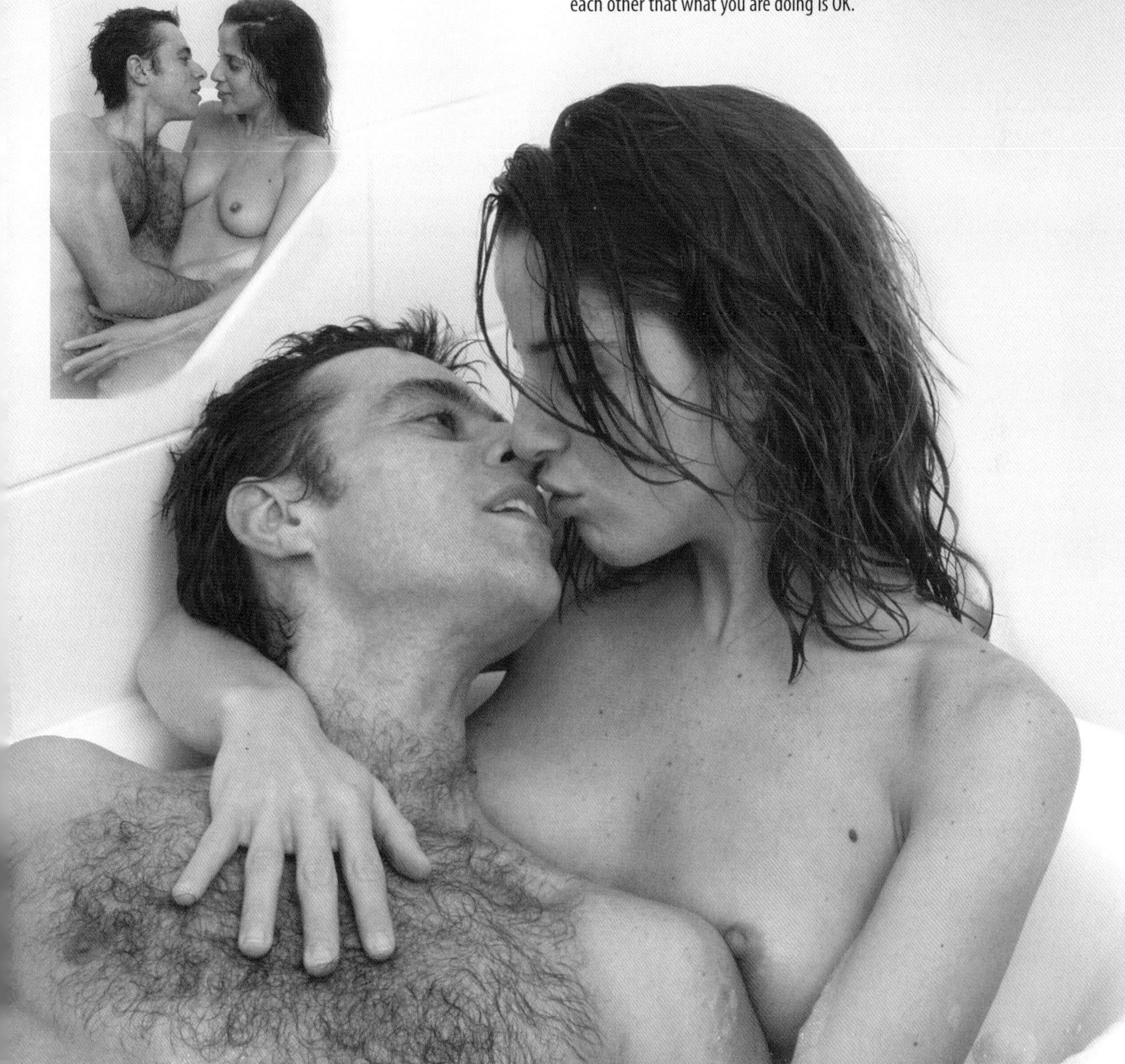

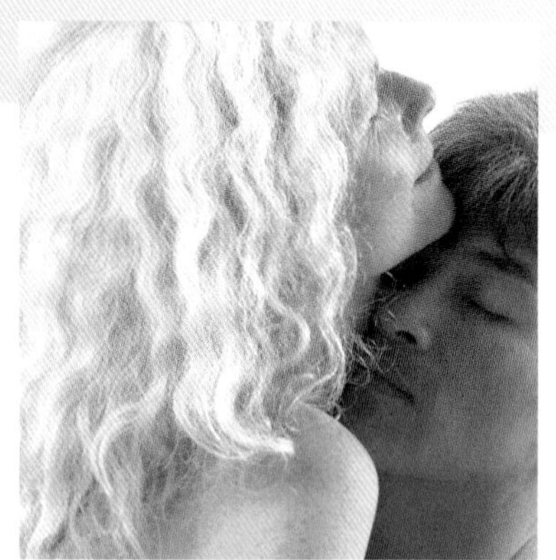

chapter 20

sexuality in the middle years

"Beautiful Melite, in the throes of middle age,
retains her youthful grace.
A blush on her cheek, she seduces with her eyes
Many years have passed
but not her girlish laughter
All the ravages of time cannot overcome true nature."
Agathias Scholasticus, Greek poet (531–580AD)

Middle age encompasses four seven-year cycles, from 42 to 69. For women, the very important transition of menopause occurs in this period. For both sexes there is a lessening of libido. But the transitions of middle age do not have to signal a decline into ill health and disability. This is a time for exploring other possibilities, to expand your potential to encompass the immense blessing this time of life can bring to you.

From 42 to 48

During this cycle, the life force energy stored in the genital area for procreation begins to become refined into wisdom. If you have lived a full and rich sexual life and have used that energy to dive deeply into love, then the transition into middle age is an experience of love expanding to include spirit. You are lifted into a new dimension of being, where everything is perceived and experienced in a lighter way. There is generally less emotional drama, life becomes more playful, and relating becomes clearer.

The transition brings an upsurge of wisdom. Sexual energy is to a certain extent reabsorbed, and can be accessed to enhance spiritual development, bringing deep inner serenity. Inner beauty becomes very important at this stage. Young people can hide their interior reality behind their outward physical appearance. But in middle age, your mind and soul are clearly visible in your face and body. Whatever you have been thinking, feeling, and doing in your life bears fruit in middle age. If you have lived in tune with your soul calling then you appear more and more radiant and people will seek you out to enjoy your presence. You become almost effervescent like a bottle of good champagne.

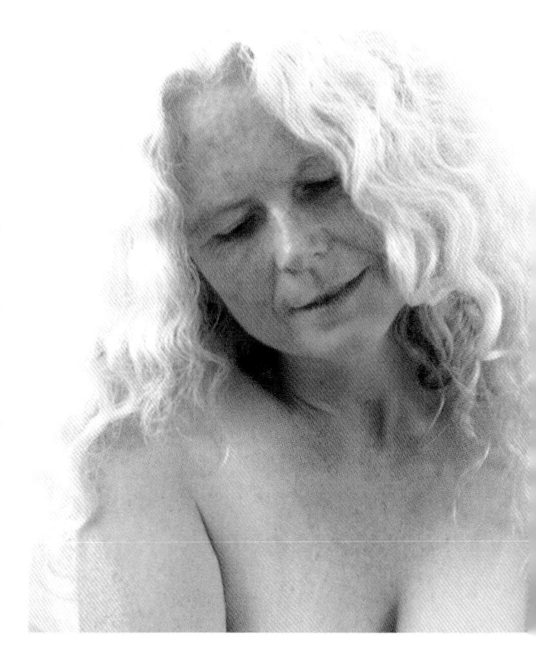

In this cycle, some women will begin to move into menopause, when the menstrual cycle comes to an end, although for others this will come in the next seven-year cycle. For an unhealthy body, menopause is a more difficult passage. If your transition into menopause and middle age is fraught with anxiety, hot flushes, depression, and other symptoms, this is a clear sign that it is time to seek holistic health care, to learn how to balance diet and hormones naturally, bringing your body back to equilibrium.

The loss of libido in this phase, for women and men, is to a certain extent a natural process. The hot passion that used to drive you to extremes in sexual behavior begins to cool. However, if you are healthy, there should be no loss of sensual pleasure. Perhaps you don't need as many genital orgasms as before. For men, perhaps your erection is not as hard, but this will not prevent you enjoying a heightened celebration of your sexual expression. At puberty, you had just one ingredient – sex. In young adulthood the ingredient of love was added, refining and heightening the pleasure. Middle age adds the ingredient of wisdom to your life's cake, making it even more delicious.

Tantra is invaluable during this life stage; it teaches ways of touching, intimacy, and celebration that expand your repertoire of sensual relating. If you rely solely on instinctual sex then you may feel very poor when your sex hormones begin to diminish. But if you learn Tantra you will feel very rich during this transition. With a free flow of energy in the body, pleasure is never lost. If your energy is in stagnation, and therefore pleasure has diminished, reclaim a free-flowing energy through healthy diet, herbs, and exercise. Touch and be touched; love and be loved.

From 48 to 55

This is the time for a step into more expansive spirituality. You may feel a deep thirst to explore meditation or prayer, to visit sacred sites, and to discover awe and wonder in your life, perhaps through a grandchild or getting closer to nature. This is a natural transformation of sexual energy into its refined potential as spiritual energy and wisdom. The same energy that used to express itself passionately in sex is now seeking other more subtle outlets. If you are a connoisseur of the delights of love, you may continue to experience sex in its most heightened aspects, where it moves into an experience of receiving grace and benediction. A couple in this state may feel that they have both dissolved as personalities and become simply love itself. A person who embraces the gift this time of life offers becomes a beacon to younger people, who find them an inspiring guide.

"The commonly held belief that ageing routinely requires pharmacological management has unfortunately led to the neglect of diet and lifestyle as the primary means to achieve healthy ageing."

From *The Okinawa Way, How To Improve Your Health and Longevity Dramatically*, Bradley Willcox MD, Craig Willcox PhD, and Makoto Suzuki MD

When a woman's time of reproduction is over, she may feel that her purpose in life is finished. This feeling can lead to depression and ill health, which may be compounded by the fact that in our society post-menopausal women are not regarded as sexually desirable. Some women even have plastic surgery to appear more youthful. Others wishing to reclaim a more youthful feeling may use synthetic hormones. This is not necessarily a bad idea, but it is wise to read the long list of possible side-effects first. A herbalist will be able to advise you about natural herbal treatments that can balance the hormone levels.

Another option is to become involved in creative endeavor during this phase. Now the possibility of making babies is over, you need to find another outlet for your creative expression. Find something to throw all your passion and energy into, to bring new surges of creativity into your life. This period of life is also a time for meditation, which will bring peace and serenity to your countenance. Inner beauty is a light that shines and illuminates the outer body with grace and radiance at any age.

A woman's capacity for sexual desire and multiple orgasms continues well into old age. Sex researchers have found that the sole factor preventing many older women from living a rich sex life is being unable to find a man to match their ardor. A man's hormone-charged libido of the younger years progressively diminishes with age. His genitals are no longer as sensitive to stimulation and he needs some days of recovery time between ejaculations. Some men use Viagra to give them an erection, but this can have side-effects. Herbs, such as Damiana, can help and are safe to use. However, during this phase the man's whole-body sensuality is awakened, and this can bring him to the most exquisite pleasure-filled states. Chinese Tantra texts recommend that older men practice the conservation of semen, so that they can continue to enjoy sex as long as they live.

Men in this age range may be very desirable to women. They may exhibit the qualities of stability, centeredness, ease, attentiveness, tenderness, and vulnerability, which are harder to find in a younger man. The mature man's mind opens up to new directions and he has more time to explore sensual delights. At this age, meditation and Tantra will help to boost a flagging libido, while also greatly enhancing serenity.

From 55 to 62

Now life energy has the opportunity to flow in a new direction. It is a time to embrace your dreams and make them a reality. Perhaps you always wanted to paint, but earning money and raising a family took precedence. During this seven-year cycle you can embrace longings or dreams with passion and joy. Allow yourself to liberate your true self on every level. You may find yourself becoming more and more child-like, casting away the burdens of responsibility and living for the moment. This is a time to dissolve boundaries and restrictions and be really free. It is almost like a new adolescence; you are writing a brand new script for yourself, born out of wisdom and experience. Some people who have always dreamed of sharing a fulfilling intimate relationship, may find that finally it is able to happen.

From 62 to 69

This is the time to let go of achievement and enter into the simplicity of just being. You are a radiance, a presence, and an inspiration, residing in grace. Your wisdom reaches a new level of maturity. You are equally able to be child-like or erudite. Sexual expression is no longer separate from love or from prayer; it is all one energy, flowing as a joyous expression into each moment. A person who has lived a life of sexual repression may at this time begin to show signs of that repressed energy bubbling up to the surface in perverted ways. Deep down they will be desperate and sad that they missed the full spectrum of life experience. It is still possible, though challenging, to catch up with yourself and make up for lost time. It is simply a matter of turning around and facing your true nature, in all its beauty and all its pain, all its longing and all its passion for life.

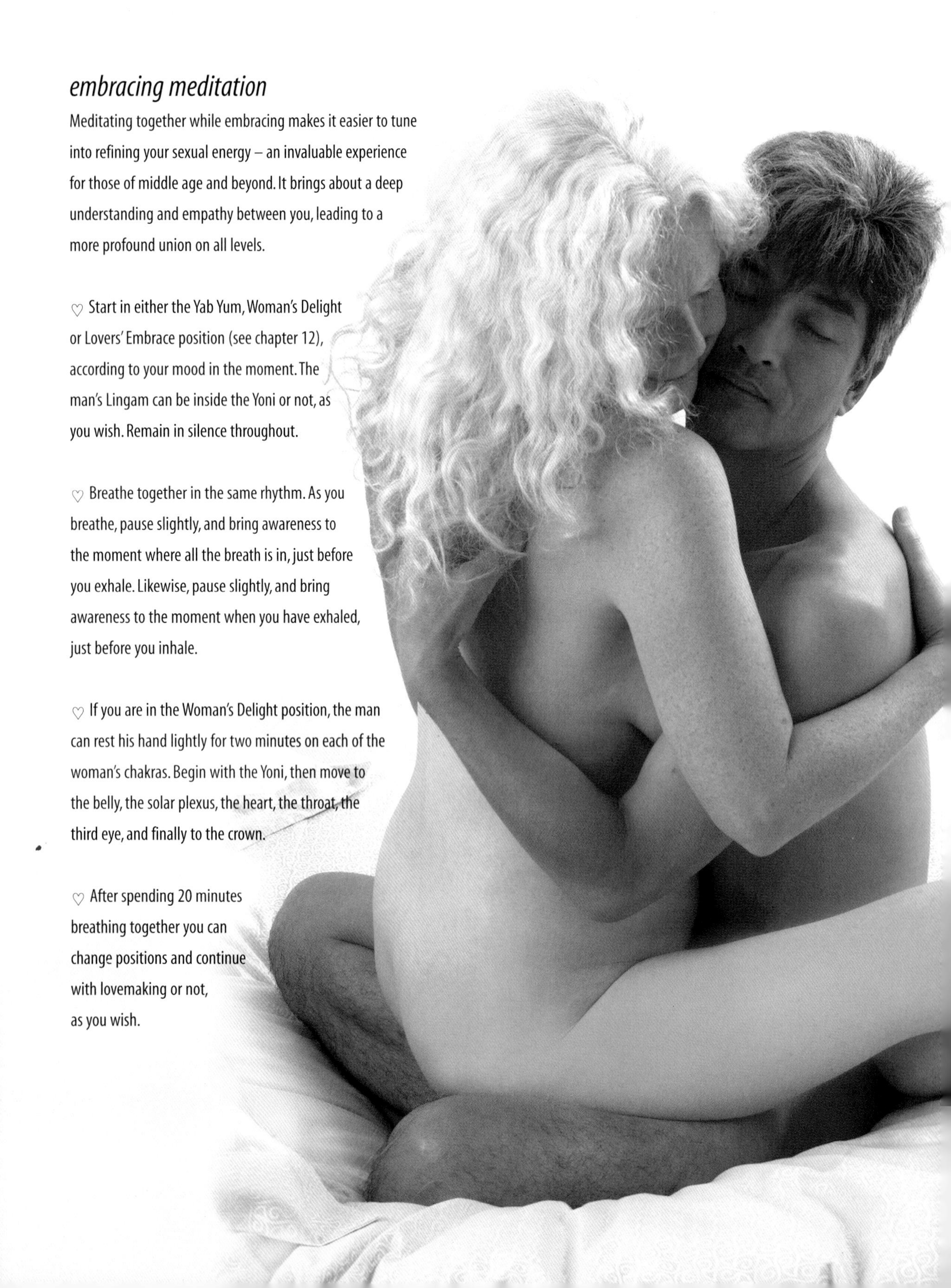

embracing meditation

Meditating together while embracing makes it easier to tune into refining your sexual energy – an invaluable experience for those of middle age and beyond. It brings about a deep understanding and empathy between you, leading to a more profound union on all levels.

♡ Start in either the Yab Yum, Woman's Delight or Lovers' Embrace position (see chapter 12), according to your mood in the moment. The man's Lingam can be inside the Yoni or not, as you wish. Remain in silence throughout.

♡ Breathe together in the same rhythm. As you breathe, pause slightly, and bring awareness to the moment where all the breath is in, just before you exhale. Likewise, pause slightly, and bring awareness to the moment when you have exhaled, just before you inhale.

♡ If you are in the Woman's Delight position, the man can rest his hand lightly for two minutes on each of the woman's chakras. Begin with the Yoni, then move to the belly, the solar plexus, the heart, the throat, the third eye, and finally to the crown.

♡ After spending 20 minutes breathing together you can change positions and continue with lovemaking or not, as you wish.

This is a first-hand account from a courageous English couple who have caught up with themselves. Les, a 58-year-old semi-retired company director, and his beloved Sally, a 45-year-old director of personal development, have embarked on a journey of self-discovery through the practice of Tantra.

Sally: When I met Les, it was a real opening, because he had done a lot of Tantra and I had grown up very proper English, in a family where you were never to show your body or express emotions. I was married for 10 years. There was no intimacy. Sex was mundane. There was a huge amount of shame. I had a yearning for sensuality and intimacy but didn't know it was my conditioning that was preventing me. For example, when Les convinced me to go to a Tantra introduction he hinted that I may be invited to remove my clothes. I jumped up and down saying "No! I will not do that!" That was three years ago. Now I am comfortable being nude on a beach.

Now, I have more sexual energy than I did in my teens, twenties or thirties. The pleasure comes in so many different ways. I can just be stroked on my back, or my hair and I let go into my pleasure, bliss, sometimes laughter, tears.

I have discovered many different types of orgasm. What is important is to be able to let go into my own energy, wherever it goes. If genital release happens, it happens. If not, no problem. What gives most pleasure is learning to dance with my own energy. To me, energy means, connecting with sensation. This may start anywhere in my body. It is like champagne. I just follow the bubbles where they want to go.

I used to be very conscious of my looks. Everything had to match. My hair had to be just so. I am now excited about the changes in my body. I even look forward to growing old. I am more and more juicy and I feel this will continue into crone-dom. We have been doing sexual healing on so many levels. Now we are really ready to begin.

Les: 16 years ago my life was at its lowest ebb, couldn't get lower. Tranquillizers and alcohol couldn't help. It became unbearable.

A complementary therapist introduced me to a man of my age who had such a shining look that I was stunned. In that moment, I said to myself, "I want what you've got. I will go anywhere, do anything, to have in myself what I see in you." Then I spent 10 years doing every kind of course I could. And things started to change. I had been 20 years in a relationship, but I left it because I was craving intimacy and couldn't find it with my partner.

On my first Tantra course I felt challenged and alive. On my second course I learned that intimacy has to start with myself. My Tantra journey is about becoming aware of myself, choosing to change, choosing to stay. I have a dance with creation by dancing with myself.

It took three years of Tantra before I could share intimacy, love, compassion, anger, sadness, orgasm, the whole beautiful range of emotions, with a woman. That is what Tantra has brought me: having permission from myself and from my partner to be who I am. To be with another who is prepared to go there. The challenge goes on – the depths, the heights. Being a good lover is about intimacy, about being totally present, intuitive, and aware – riding the wave, being selfish and selfless dancing with what is. If you want good sex, create a loving, caring, nurturing relationship. If you don't have that, you can't have good sex.

On a purely practical level, I am 58, not 18. What happens to my energy when I ejaculate now is different. I lose interest in a sexual space for around 3 to 8 days. Living with a Tantric woman 14 years my junior is quite challenging. If I am making love and being with Tantric energy, having full-body orgasm, or orgasm just with the little finger, I am building my sexual energy. By using Tantra methods, including retention of ejaculation, to build the energy, erection is not a problem at all. I often feel the same degree of sexual energy as when I was 20.

chapter 21

sensuality for elders

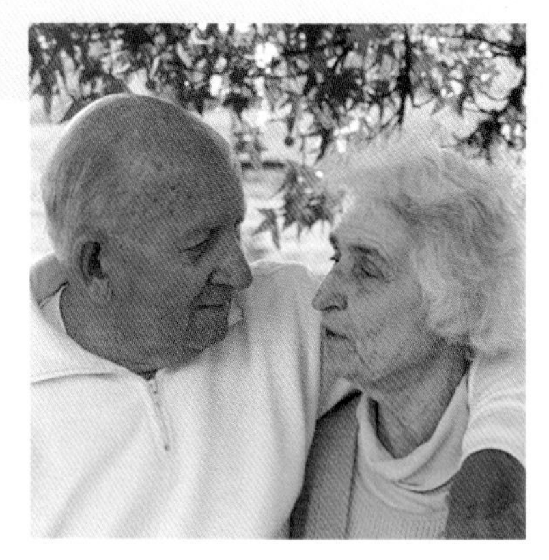

"Even clothed in wrinkles, dear Philinna
you are more beautiful than the young
I'd sooner taste the apples
hanging heavy from your boughs
than pinch the firm breasts of girls
I've no taste for the young
Your autumn outshines a mortal spring
your winter warmer than a summer sun."
Paulus Silentiarius, 6th century AD

Okinawa, in Japan, has the longest living population yet found (where birth records can be traced, proving individuals' longevity). At 100 years plus, Okinawans may be still working in the garden, taking other forms of exercise, travelling, or even having sex, with their brains and bodies functioning perfectly. A 25-year study has found that their radiant health has nothing to do with genetic disposition or region, and everything to do with eating habits, exercise, and outlook on life. Oyakawasan, who went fishing to celebrate his 105th birthday, says: "It is important . . . to enjoy life . . . and to get a good night's sleep. One should not be concerned with little things or worry about age or appearance, or complain about the body's natural aches and pains . . . One must focus on the good things in life . . . and remember to smile."

The last phase of life is in resonance with the ultimate human attributes: love, compassion, wisdom, and spiritual awakening. These attributes may shine forth like flowers in a well-tended garden, or they may be hidden under a jungle of undergrowth. How this phase is experienced depends entirely on how you have lived your life up to this time. It is like standing on a high hill, looking back over your life path. Either this sight will bring joy and fulfilment, for a life well lived, or sorrow, for a zigzag path with many mistaken turns. One elderly man, when questioned about his life said, "My message to young people would be, do what I should have done, not what I did do."

This life phase contains several possibilities of seven-year cycles: 69–76, 76–83, 83–90, and so on. Each cycle carries within it the possibility of life moving into the transition of death, and so carries within itself the question, "Have I fulfilled my life purpose, or is there still something to learn, to share, and to develop?" When the life purpose is fulfilled, or when a person comes to feel that no more evolution is possible in this life, then the physical body is not needed, and the soul rejoins spirit beyond matter.

It is the quality of a life that is truly important, not its length. Old age need not mean ill health, hospital, and inevitably a home for the dying. It is possible to live a healthful and happy life right up to the moment of death. The idea that disease indiscriminately attacks innocent victims takes away people's inclination to search for causes in their lifestyle and environment. To discover the secret of health, take a profound look at your attitude and lifestyle. Without healthful longevity, a fulfilling sensuality for the elderly is not so easy.

Respect for elders

In aboriginal societies and eastern cultures, traditionally elders have been tremendously respected and seen as the guardians of wisdom born out of life experience. In oral traditions, it may have taken almost a whole lifetime to learn the thousands of years of wisdom passed down through previous generations, which was carried like a priceless treasure by the elderly. Those seeds of wisdom were then passed on, ensuring a continuity of the dignity of the people. Learning from their ancestors' lessons meant that they didn't repeat their ancestors' mistakes, and could benefit from their ancestors' discoveries, so each generation became wiser than the last. Young people naturally turned toward the elderly like young plants toward the sun, receiving the full benefit of the wisdom of a lifetime. Because of this, old age was not something to be feared, but a time to reap the rewards of a life well lived. The elderly were respected, loved, and seen as a role model by the younger generation.

Spiritual wisdom intensifies with old age, and the elders were more likely to be able to offer healing or spiritual benediction. In India, it was thought that old age was the best time to leave the world and move toward a life of meditation and spirituality. The proximity of death means that many worldly concerns begin dropping away, as you come closer and closer to the light of the spirit. It is in old age that you sense your angel as a continuous guiding presence. In the face of a beloved old person, the younger generation can sense a sublime detachment, a love that transcends space and time. These qualities can be cultivated and enhanced through the regular practice of meditation.

tips for healthful longevity

- ♡ A balanced diet that gives nourishment rather than toxins to the body
- ♡ A sense of humor
- ♡ A continuing curiosity to learn
- ♡ A strong sense of creative purpose
- ♡ Gentle and regular exercise such as walking, dancing, Tai Chi or Yoga
- ♡ An attunement to the divine through meditation or prayer
- ♡ A sense of involvement with community

Sensual aliveness

Ageing couples often suffer from impotence and loss of interest in sex. However, while the physical causes of erectile and libido disorders become more prevalent with age, most such problems have a psychological basis. If a person's libido diminishes, they may become depressed and therefore avoid sexual relations. However, Tantra can transform sex from a solely reproductive urge into an art for giving birth to an ongoing inner ecstasy, which is not dependent on the reproductive organs. If you cultivate the art of sexual ecstasy through Tantra, when nature begins to withdraw its emphasis on reproduction you will be able to slip out of that identity easily, with no loss of sensual aliveness.

"When I became old, my own death stared me in the face too boldly to ignore. So I walked with it, holding its hand, until one day it was no more and my hand was empty. Since that moment clarity has come. I love old age. I love the twilight. I know that I shall love the darkness."

Archan

In sexual exploration at this stage of life, there is a discrepancy between men and women. Women tend to live 5–8 years longer than men, so an elderly woman choosing a lover is wise to go for a younger man. Another discrepancy is that a man's hormonally based sexuality reaches a peak at age 18, then slowly decreases throughout life. So an older man has less erection capability and also less of an urge to ejaculate. However, if he has cultivated his all-over body sensitivity, he will express his love in many tender ways, bringing a wealth of erotic possibilities to a sensual union. Freed of the lust of youth, love play can be a delightful journey of discovery and play, similar to the highly tantalizing and nourishing kissing and caressing of young adolescents. If meditation is brought to it, this love play can take on the quality of eternity, which transcends physical limitations. Also, if a man has learned the practice of retention of ejaculation, he can continue to enjoy lovemaking with more vigor and more possibility of erection.

love in winter

I have loved the crescent moon at twilight
I have loved an oak-wood fire on a night of rain
I have loved your voice, speaking softly in the dark–
I have loved such simple things –
It may be, in the time we were together –
So long ago that not a trace remains,
Those very things I love now,
I loved then.

Kay

An older woman, depending on the state of her health, is able to continue to experience sexual arousal in all its phases, even including multiple orgasm. She may not feel the same drive to pursue her desire as she did in her younger years, but the vitality of her libido remains intact. Some women experience a gradual diminishing of their vaginal juiciness and with it a complete loss of libido. This is a sign that hormone levels have dropped below a healthy balance; it can be remedied through natural herbal remedies, healthful diet, and exercise.

Libido does not necessarily mean being hot and horny. It may mean a delicious all-over body sensuality, where you feel pleasure in many aspects of life. This sensuous energy may like to be expressed through sexual play, or through other creative acts in life. Just follow what brings delight to you and go on enhancing that in any way possible.

keep attentive on the fire

This Tantra meditation helps to renew and rejuvenate the life force. Practice it regularly, for a few weeks or more, and you will notice an increase in your energy.

> "At the start of sexual union
> keep attentive on the fire
> in the beginning,
> and so continuing,
> avoid the embers in the end."
>
> Shiva Sutra

♡ During lovemaking, as sensual, sexual energy begins building, just stay with that delicious sensuality, without seeking peak energy or orgasm. If there is penetration, keep the movements soft and flowing. Do not be goal-oriented, simply enjoy the moment.

♡ Keeping a sense of playfulness and joy will recharge the life force of both partners, creating a circle of energy. Aim to stay in this playful space for around 40 minutes. Then lie silently in each other's arms for another 20 minutes.

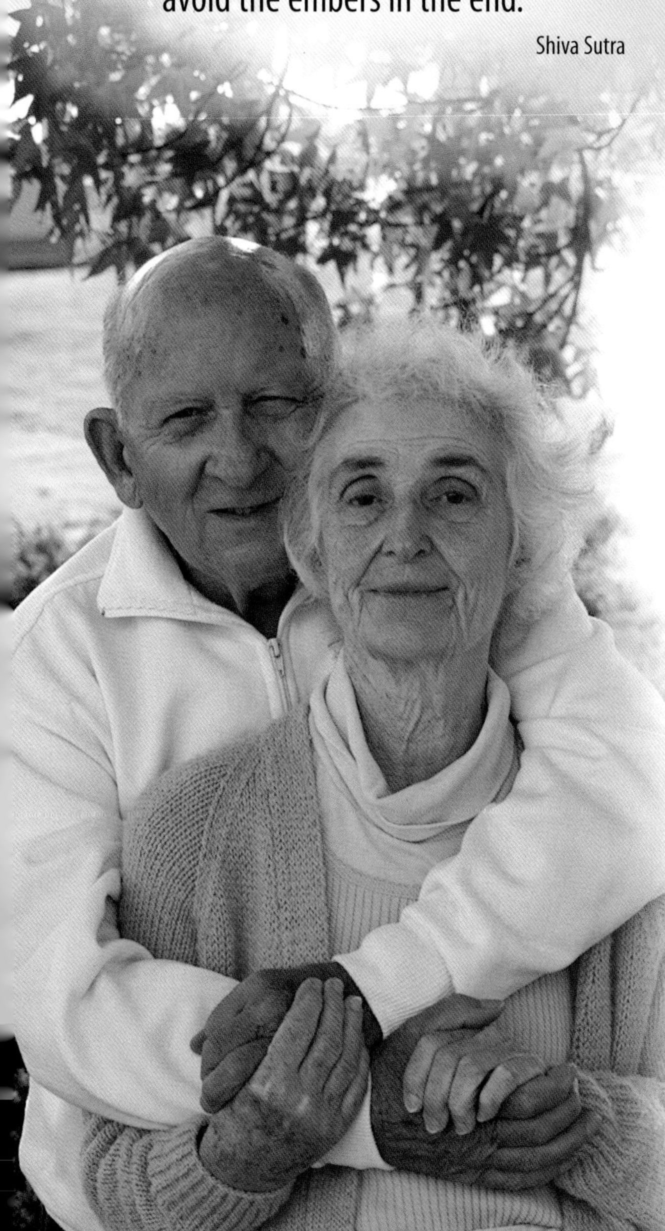

Al (77) and Kay (84) are from Oregon, USA. He is a photographer who loves to capture on film "the beauty of the world". His wife of 30 years died a couple of years before he met Kay, "the love of his life". Kay, a writer, has seven children, ten grandchildren, and four great-grandchildren. Her husband of 30 years died two years before she met Al.

Kay: We feel we were together in another life. When we came together as lovers, it was not as strangers, it was a reunion. I astonished myself by whispering "You are my bliss" when he embraced me.
Al: We have learned to drop all inhibitions, leave them aside. Everything else comes naturally.
Kay: When we throw off our clothes and jump into bed, it is as if we have simultaneously thrown off all inhibition and self-judgements. We try new things, learning about each other. Our bodies have lost the attractions of youth. Age has had its way with us, and there are battle scars. But our souls have grown rich and full. When we make love, soul and body are one.

Our advice to other elderly people is: respect and treasure your partner, accept with gratitude what you are given, and every touch and caress will be beautiful. Forget the inhibitions, forget the past. Get to know each other like two happy youngsters, free of guilt, free of regrets. Live in the moment.

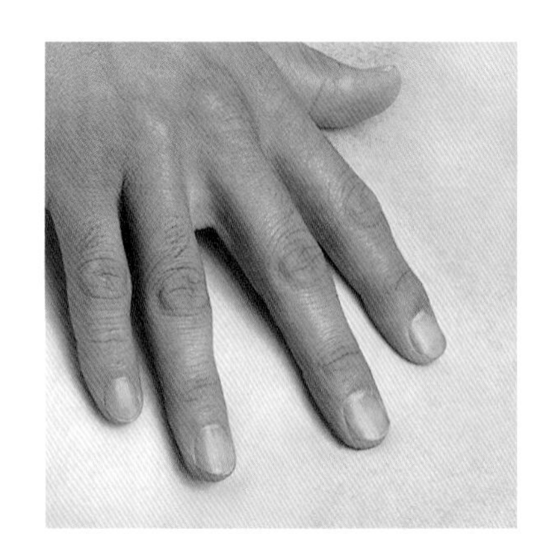
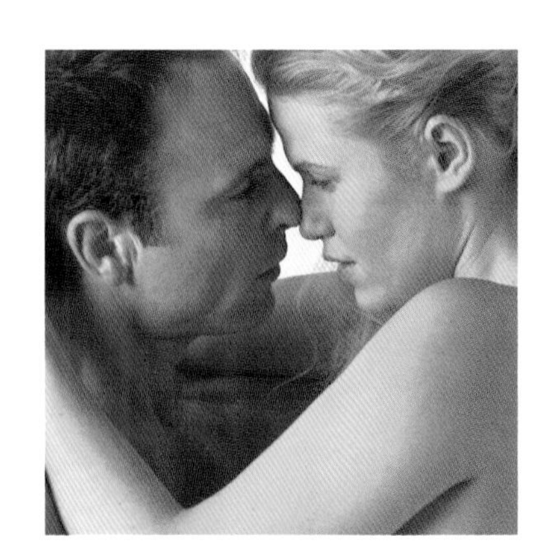
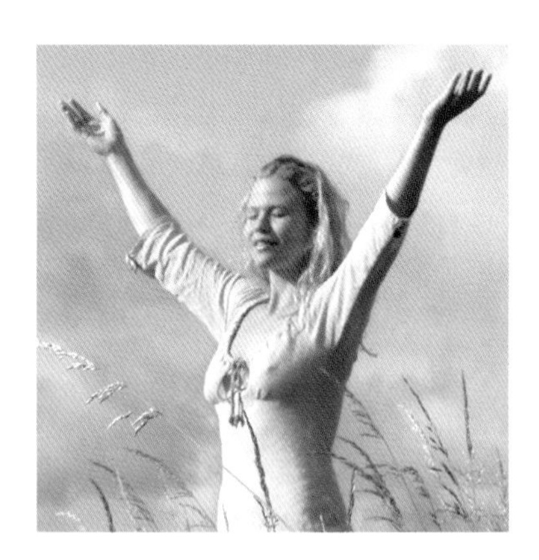
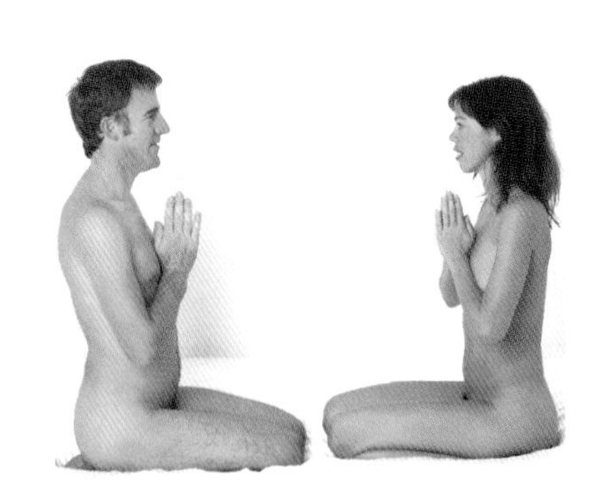
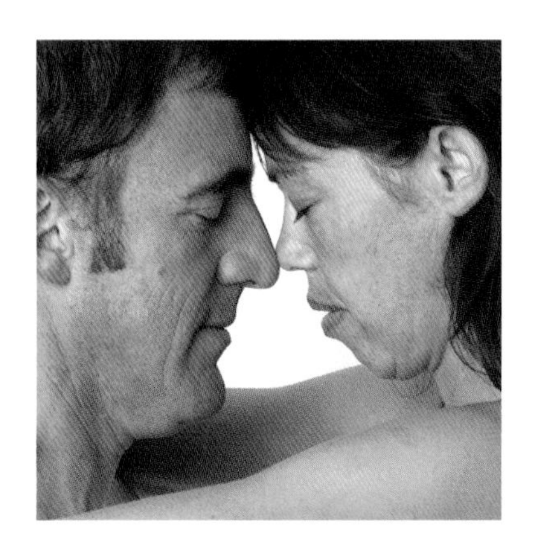
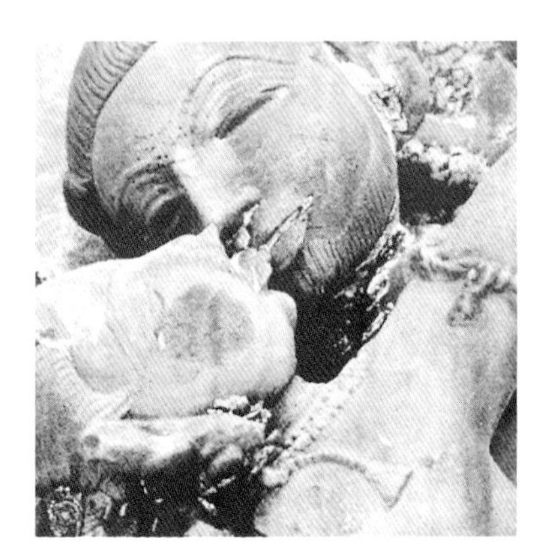

part 6
fulfilment

The search for fulfilment can appear like a maze. We may become lost in the myriad twists and turns of life, and so not discover the path leading to the center. The maze is rather like a Zen koan – a riddle whose solution can only be found by entering into a state of higher consciousness. In this state, suddenly we have a bird's eye view of the maze of life, love, and sexuality.

The state of higher consciousness is not something separate from us, to be attained through effort. It is more a remembering to come back home to who we are in our sensual aliveness. The secret for discovering this homecoming is practicing meditation, thus heightening awareness and sensitivity. A sensitive and aware person has inner knowing, through being connected to the source of life, aware of an interconnectedness with all dimensions of being.

In this discovery, we can benefit from the transformative research carried out by the Tantra mystics of ages past. They may inspire our steps forward, into a new dawn of Tantra, where the art of love is placed in the highest esteem, transforming each individual and society as a whole.

chapter 22

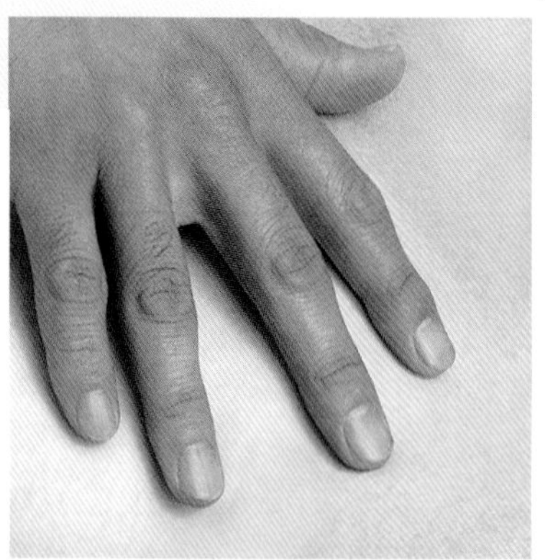

the senses in sex play

"All of us in different ways
Think of God
Beyond senses and feelings
And yet it is only
In the essence of loving
That God is found"
song from the Baul Mystics, of Bengal, India,
translated by D Battacharya

Sensitivity means both your response to stimulation of the senses, and a heightened awareness of yourself and others in personal relationships. When your sensitivity is awakened, your experience of life is enhanced in all dimensions. Through the senses you see, hear, feel, smell, and taste the world around you. And also through your senses you can enter into a subjective experience of happiness and orgasmic pleasure. If your senses become dull, you are more likely to become sad and depressed. As you enhance your sensitivity, you discover spontaneous delight. Your inner and outer world sparkle with aliveness.

Each sense organ functions like a swing door. In one direction it opens to physical pleasure or pain, while in the other it opens to an expansion of the soul and spiritual awareness. The more you expand your sensory awareness, the greater is your spiritual awakening.

During love play with or without a partner, focusing on the different senses can expand your capacity for sensual awakening, both physical and spiritual. In this way you enhance your total life experience to its maximum potential.

Each sense can give pain or pleasure. Many people deaden their senses in response to traumatic experiences or conditioning that inspire fear of being truly alive. So it can happen that as you enter on a journey to awaken your sensitivity, you find yourself also re-living and releasing memories of times when for protection you have chosen to cut yourself off from one or more of your senses. As these memories are released, you may experience strong emotions. It is very healthy to allow this emotional release. If you experience anger, beat a punch bag or large cushion and let the anger out – try roaring like a lion. Afterward, just sit silently for a few minutes and discover how alive and flowing your energy has become. If sadness wells up, let the tears flow. Tears function like stormy weather, clearing the air and giving rise to an opening of the heart and a deeper insight into life. If you can cry in the arms of your lover, it brings deep intimacy.

Once you have released whatever was holding you back from being fully alive, you may experience a sudden burst of joyous expansion and pleasure. The message from your body and soul is: fulfilment is possible if you are willing to open up and expand your sensitivity on all levels. Our natural state of being is bliss. Allowing an expansion of sensory awareness will lead you slowly but surely toward a life where even a simple act such as breathing becomes ecstatic.

The exercises on pages 156–61 present simple methods for opening and enhancing each sense.

"I had thought that sensory awareness would be mainly about massage and touch, but actually it seems to have satisfied some deep need in me to be more in touch with every aspect of myself and in tune with the rhythm of life."

Valerie, Tantra group participant

"We have tasted the vibrations of love, licked the sensuality, touched the sacred, danced the universal sounds, sung the emotion of the heart, and tamed the light."

Anne-France, Tantra group participant

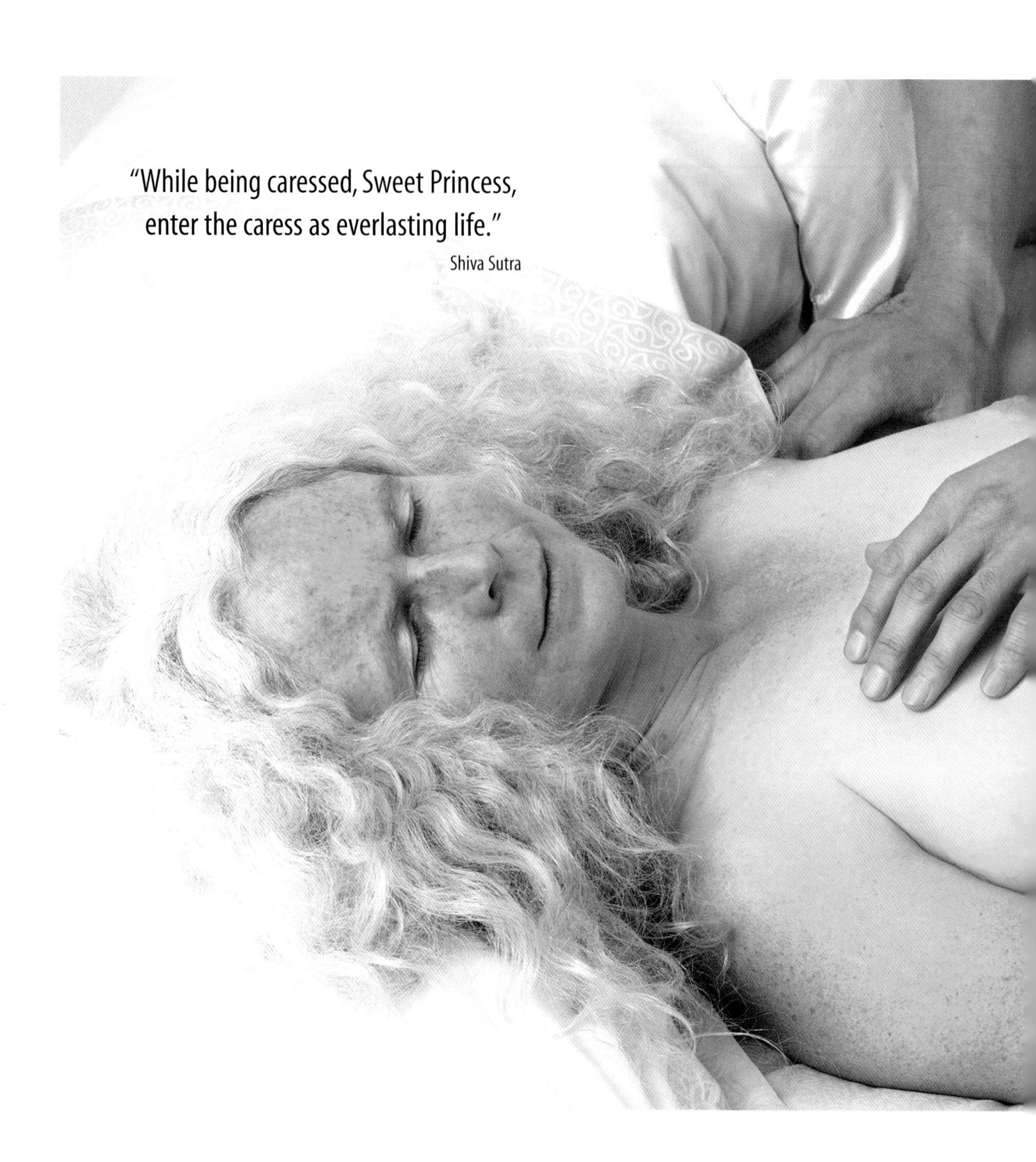
"While being caressed, Sweet Princess,
enter the caress as everlasting life."
Shiva Sutra

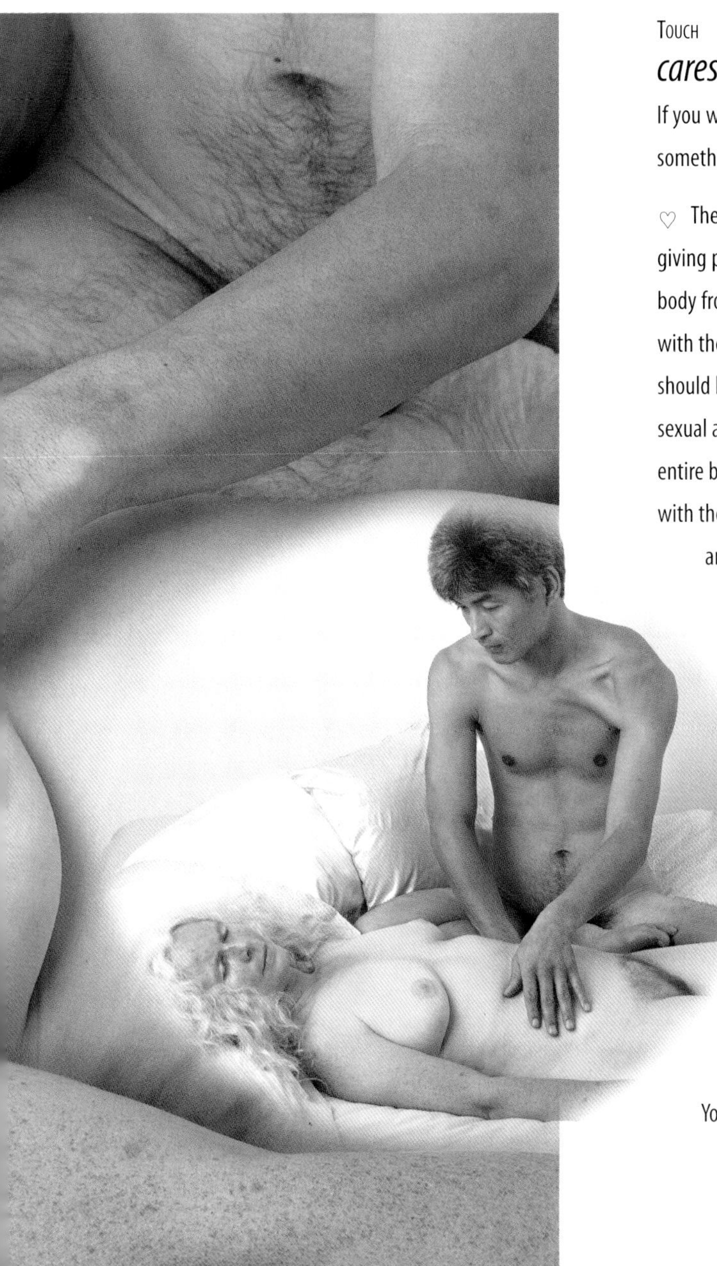

Touch

caressing meditation

If you would like music to accompany this meditation, choose something very soft, sweet, and melodic.

♡ The receiving partner lies down naked on her front. The giving partner sits next to her and gently caresses the receiver's body from head to toe. Use only one hand at a time, touching mainly with the fingertips and moving slowly and smoothly. Your touch should be light, but not so light that it tickles. It is not trying to bring sexual arousal, but rather an awakening of sensitivity throughout the entire body. The receiver should focus on the present moment, staying with the experience of pleasurable touch. This caress brings pleasure, and at the same time deep relaxation, allowing the receiver to enter a state of expanded consciousness through heightened sensitivity.

♡ After 10 minutes, ask the receiver to turn over to lie on her back. Caress her front, from head to toe for a further 10 minutes. After the caress, sit silently by your partner's side, leaving her in her own space for a few minutes.

♡ The receiver remains silent throughout the experience. To create the right mood, the giver can repeat the Shiva Sutra (left) from time to time.

♡ Exchange roles and repeat the caressing meditation. You may wish to follow the meditation with lovemaking.

a meal you will never forget

♡ Prepare a sensuous meal, to include a variety of tastes and scents. Because you will be opening your senses of taste and smell to a heightened degree, it is best to use only freshly prepared food, not packaged or frozen, and without additives. Curry or other spicy foods are ideal. Avoid garlic, since its anaesthetic qualities lower sensitivity, and its strong smell and taste will over-ride everything else. Include a good wine or other quality drink.

♡ Allow yourselves enough time to luxuriate in the experience.

♡ Blindfold your partner and seat him comfortably so that he can recline if he wishes. Feed him very slowly and sensuously, allowing him plenty of time to smell and taste each mouthful. Use your fingers or a fork, as you wish. The receiver may make sounds of appreciation as he enters deeper into a heightened awareness of eating. From time to time, you may wish to whisper the Shiva Sutra (below) for this meditation into his ear.

♡ You can also practice this method naked, which will enhance the creativity of the experience. Bellies make excellent plates, and dessert never tastes better than when licked from a Lingam, a breast, or a Yoni. Wine drunk from the lips of a lover is nectar of the gods.

♡ You can feed your partner the whole meal before you exchange roles, or you can take turns for around 10 minutes at a time.

♡ To practice this alone, prepare your meal and sit naked, serving yourself with your hands. Chew very slowly with your eyes closed, savoring every mouthful.

"When eating or drinking, become the taste of food or drink, and be filled."

Shiva Sutra

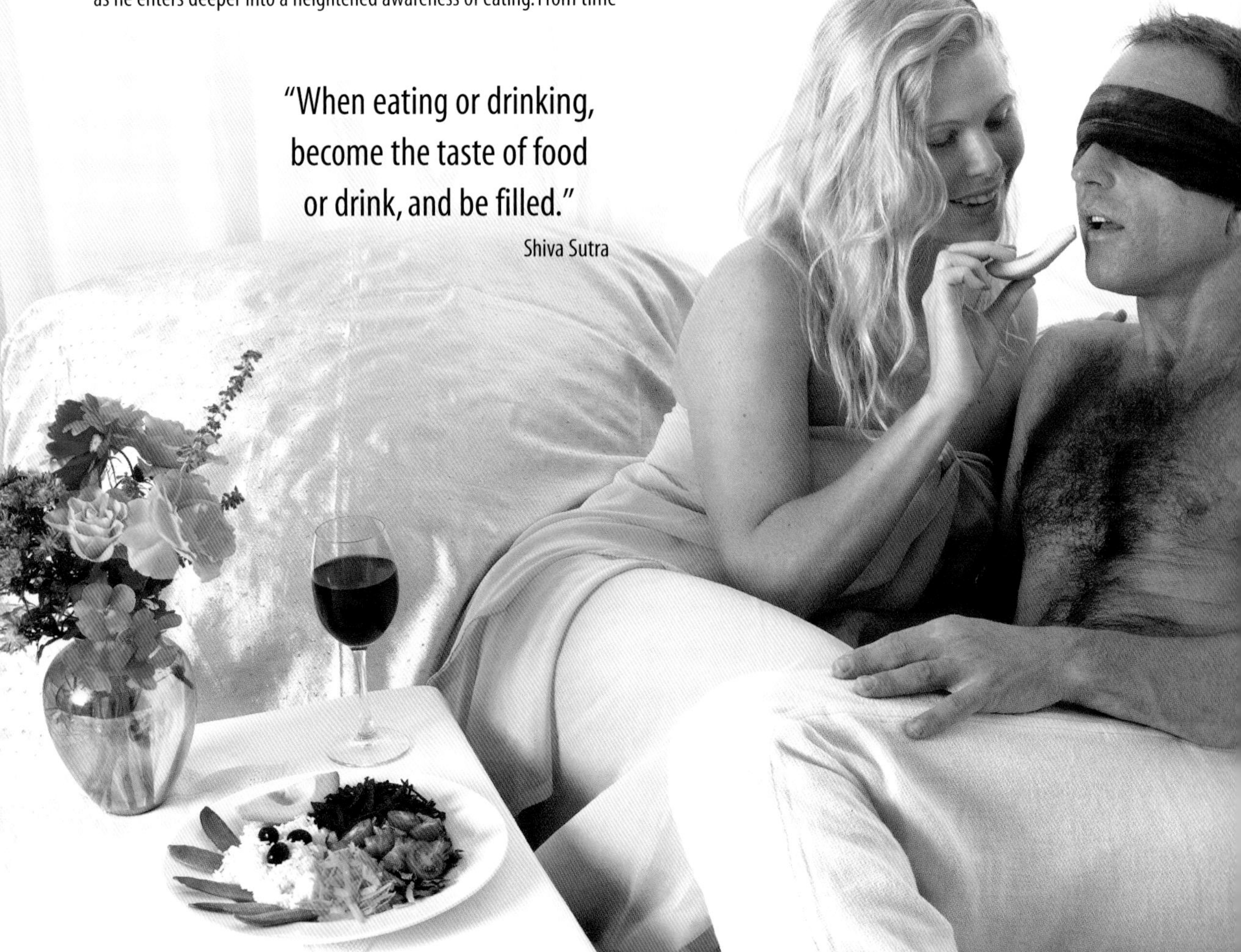

looking with the eyes of love

This meditation links the eyes with the heart. In it you reverse the normal process of *looking at* to *receptive vision*.

♡ Sit facing your partner, looking into each other's eyes, for about 10 minutes. Simply receive your partner's look. This way of seeing is called Yin vision. It creates receptivity, and opens right brain function. When the right brain is activated it enhances feelings of love, and when love is present you will discover the blessings inherent in what you are seeing.

♡ You can also try this during lovemaking.

♡ To practice this alone, look into your own eyes in a mirror for about 5 minutes. This is Yang or outward vision. Then allow the eyes in the mirror to look into you for a further 5 minutes, using Yin or receptive vision. Next look at a tree or a flower for 5 minutes. Then allow the tree or flower to look into you for 5 minutes.

♡ In both these exercises, using Yang vision first, and then Yin vision, allows you to appreciate the contrast between them.

"Look lovingly at some object. Do not go to another object.
Here in the middle of the object – the blessing."

Shiva Sutra

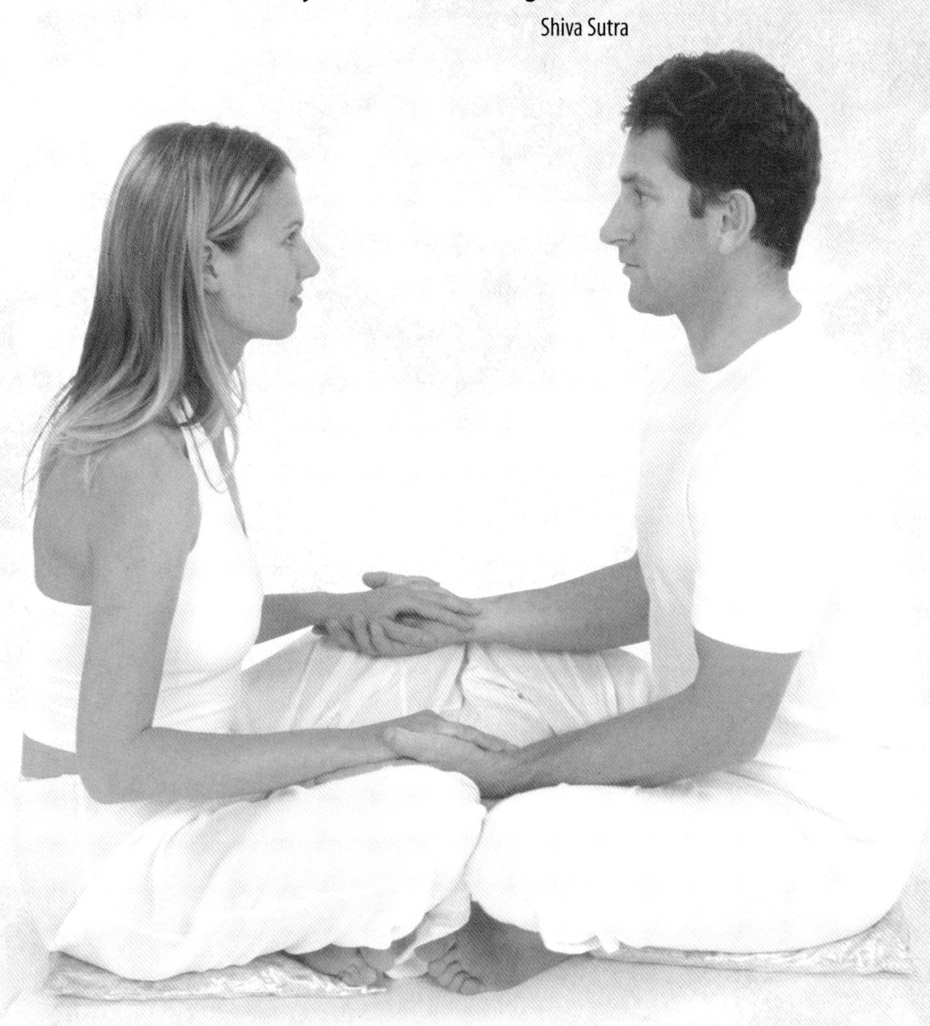

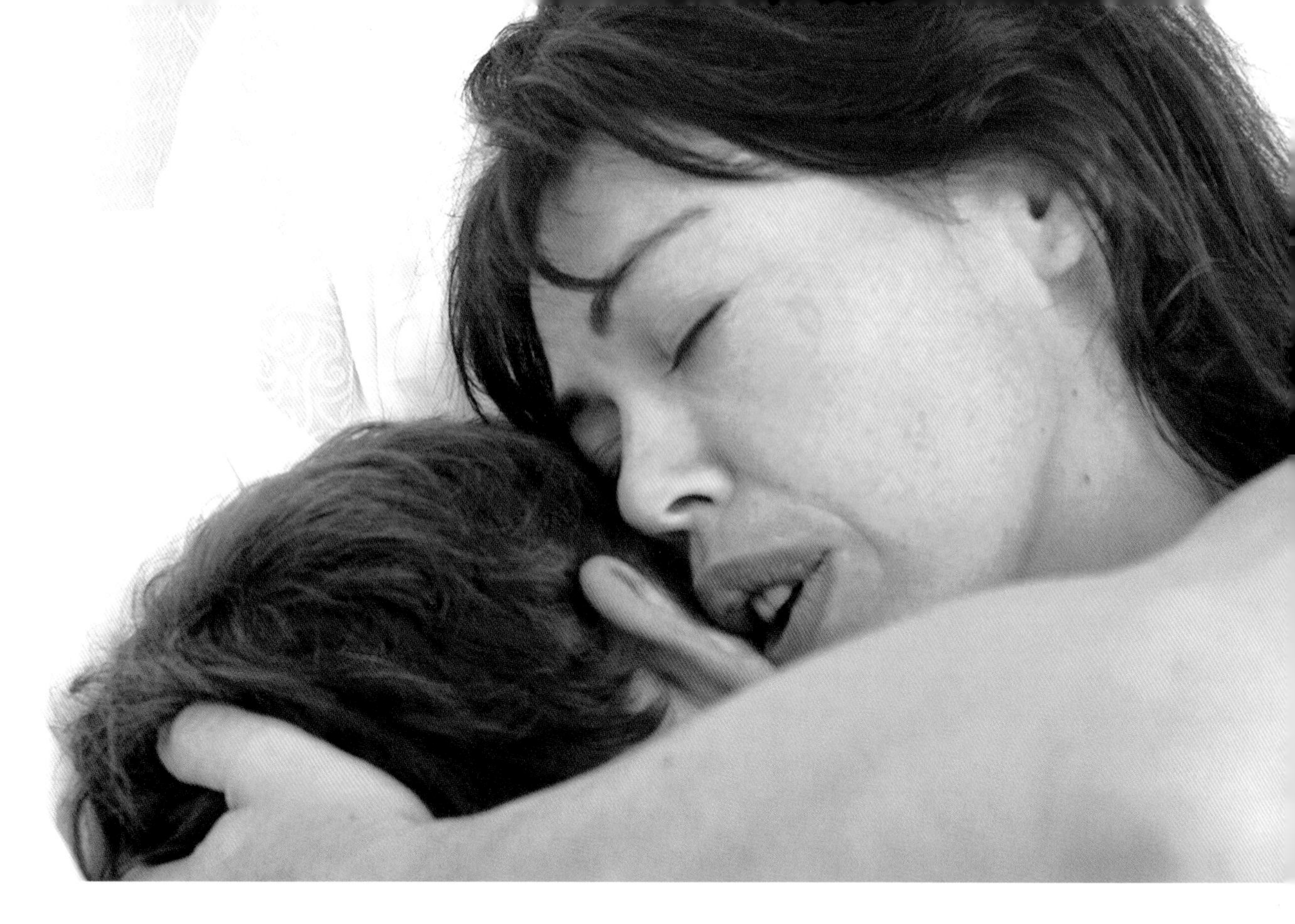

Hearing

uncensored lovemaking

This is a very simple method, but it may take courage to practice it. Both partners need to agree to it *before* making love.

♡ While making love, both partners tell each other whatever is happening, moment by moment, without censorship. In lovemaking there are many sensations, experiences, longings, and moods which pass by in rapid succession. Allow yourself to express it all.

♡ This is not a conversation – both partners may speak at the same time. Also it is not a time to judge and blame your partner. Focus on your own personal sensory experience moment by moment, as it relates to your shared sensations during sexual union. You can also express passions, longings, poetry, laughter, and tears – anything that is connected to the present moment.

♡ Generally, a lot of feelings are locked up and unexpressed during lovemaking. This creates inhibition, so the sex act may not have a chance to be as marvellously freeing as it could be. With this method, you throw inhibitions to the wind, through speaking your truth in an impassioned, shared experience.

♡ If you enjoy the experience, repeat it seven times for deeper transformation. After seven times your ability for a deep truthful communication will be established.

♡ To practice this alone, use this method while self-pleasuring. Make sure to speak out loud, for if you speak only internally it will not have the same impact. Cry, laugh, tell yourself how beautiful you are, how sexy you are, and how much you love yourself. Just go on and on expressing what is there, without inhibition.

four-minute laughing meditation

Some Tibetan monks use this method in their monasteries and it is a great way to start the day. Since laughter enhances your immune function, it is very good for health and longevity. It will also help to make you more orgasmic.

Seriousness can be considered as a disease, because it makes the whole world look dull and heavy. There is a saying: "Laugh, and the world laughs with you. Cry, and you cry alone." Laughter transforms your life, helping you to transcend illusions and to come close to the source of creation, the cosmic joke in which we are all participants.

Use this meditation every morning for 21 days to experience its full impact on your life. Afterward, you may choose to continue for a longer period, or just use it now and again.

♡ When you wake up in the morning, before you open your eyes, spend one minute stretching like a cat, allowing your whole body to give a great yawn.

♡ Laugh from your belly, moving into a whole body experience. Laugh loudly for three minutes.

♡ Open your eyes and begin your day.

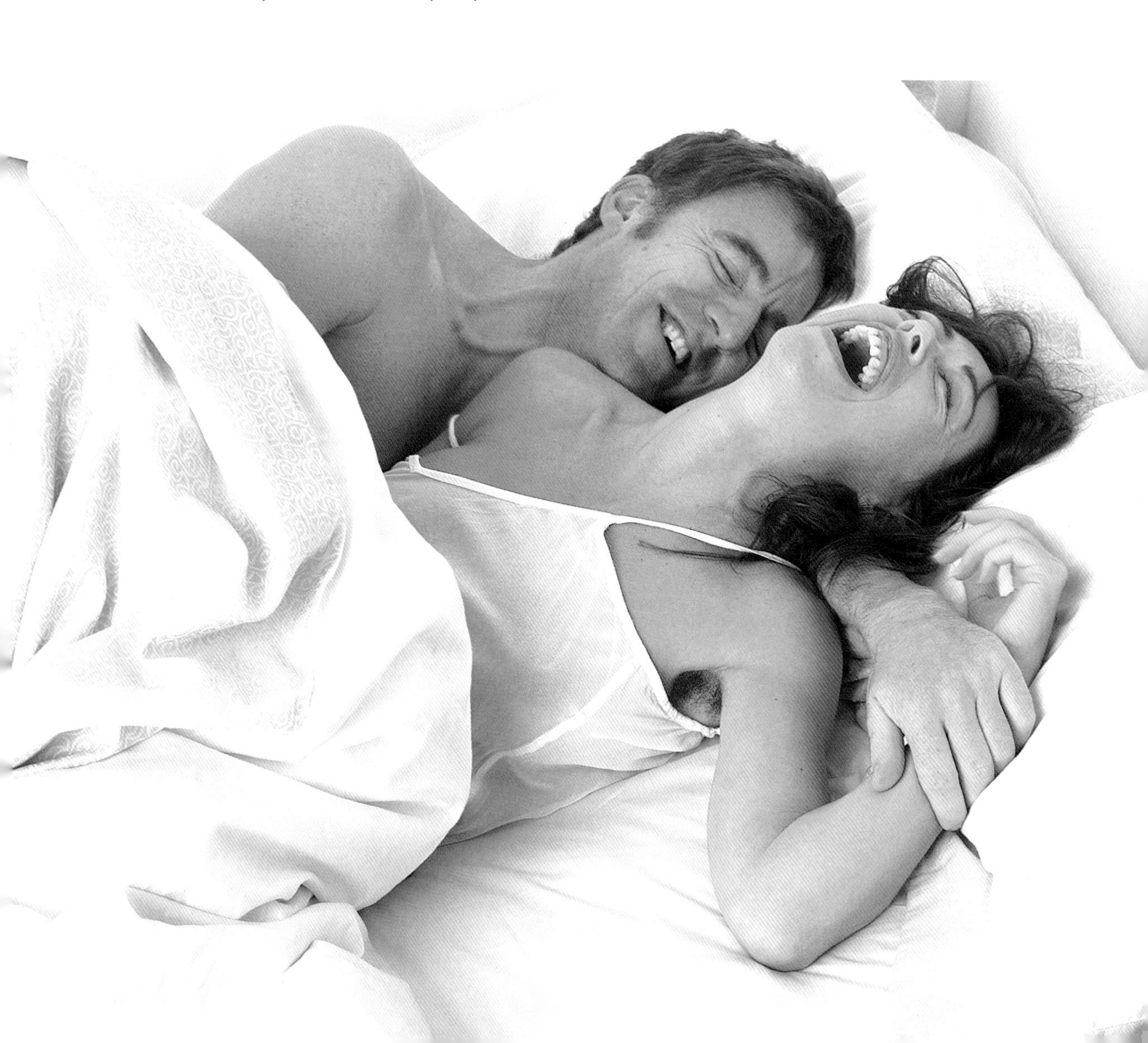

chapter 23

communication between lovers

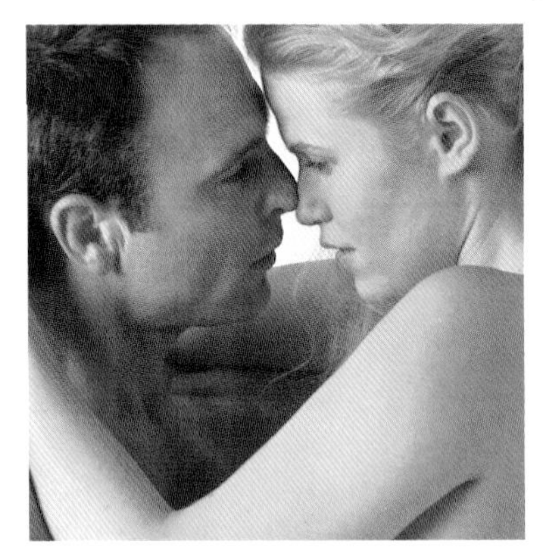

"What is it men in women do require?
The lineaments of Gratified Desire.
What is it women do in men require?
The lineaments of Gratified Desire."
From *The Notebook* (1793) William Blake

To have open, rich, and nurturing communication between lovers is a delicate art. It requires a sincere desire to know love in its fullness. A true communication will bring about communion, where both feel seen, understood, loved, and at one with the other. You may wonder how this can be possible between two such diverse beings as man and woman. We can say from our own experience that it is possible. And we have also seen it happen with couples we have worked with. Therefore, we know it is possible for everyone.

When you let go into love, you are surrendering – not to the personality of your partner but to love itself. By its very nature, the state of being in love with another human being asks you to let go, be receptive, and surrender. The mistake many couples make is to think that they have to surrender to their partner's personality, which is usually what your ego clashes against. The personality is actually a mask we hold up to the world, which is full of false pretensions designed to hide our vulnerability. Naturally, people become quite squeamish at the thought of saying "yes" to this mask. There are times when your whole being wants to rebel against it. However, beyond the personality is the principle of love itself, which has no name and no form, yet permeates all. If you can allow yourself to go a step deeper, and surrender to that love principle, you may gain a very different view of your partner. He or she will become the conduit through which you can experience infinite love.

The ten tips on pages 163–5 will help you to build deep and nourishing communication with your partner.

ten tips for deeper communication

1) Look at your partner with receptive Yin vision (see page 159). When couples are newly in love they feel totally in tune with each other. We may say this is because they are wearing "rose-tinted glasses" – rose is a color associated with love. New lovers spontaneously move into Yin vision without realizing it. Using it consciously will open your heart to love – the great healer that gives rise to understanding, compassion, and fulfilment. This is a good way to begin any type of communication.

2) When discussing delicate subjects, try to use the word "I". "You" easily carries blame with it, and a whole world of projection in its wake. If there is any blame, judgement, or condemnation in your words, your partner will close down to protect themselves. From that point, the flow of communication stops. However, when you use the word "I", this turns the arrow back toward yourself, and you can use it to expose the roots of your vulnerability around an issue.

An example of using the word "I" may run something like this: instead of saying, "You hurt me," say, "I am hurting." Close your eyes and explore the roots of this hurt – chances are this pattern of feeling hurt has been there a very long time. Uncover the first memory associated with it and describe it, aloud. By exposing its roots in this way, magically the issue no longer carries the same emotional charge. You are free to be more spontaneous and in the moment with life energy; instead of reacting, you will now be able to respond.

When one partner has the courage to expose their vulnerability, the other partner will automatically, and in every case, feel a welling up of love and understanding, and will in turn open their heart. Blame is a defence weapon, and using it leaves both partners closed and self-protective. Exposure, on the other hand, leads to openness, and through this communion becomes possible.

3) Be the first one to open. Often, both partners are playing the same protection game: "I will open myself and expose my vulnerability only if my partner does it first". The fear of opening is simply the fear of exposing wounds and vulnerability, having no defence, and so perhaps getting hurt. This fear stems from childhood, when you were vulnerable and dependent. When you consciously decide to open as an adult you are taking responsibility for yourself, choosing to embrace all that life has to offer, and grow through it. Openness and vulnerability become empowering and liberating. Love means having the courage to expose your wounds to your lover, who functions as a mirror to help you expand into healing and wisdom.

4) If you have anger that would like to overflow on to your partner, choose to express it on a pillow instead. There is nothing wrong with anger. It is simply pure life force energy, which finds no outlet and so explodes like a volcano. Do not judge yourself about your anger, just find a healthy way to express it. Exploding on to your partner creates unnecessary wounding. Exploding on to a pillow wounds no one, clears the air, and creates fresh new levels of creative energy.

Each household should have a punch-bag or a fat red cushion for releasing anger. Just kneel down in front of it and really let go, beat it, throttle it, scream and shout at it. Then close your eyes and sit silently in front of it for 5 minutes, using that time to let the turbulence settle into a witnessing of body, mind, and emotions. With this method, you break the chain of inflicting violence and abuse one on another.

5) When you would like to share something, remember to share from your heart. If you cut yourself off from your heart as a means of protection, and speak only from your head, you can easily create a very charged atmosphere. If you say your truth from your heart, no matter what that truth is, it is impossible to wound the other. The heart, as the home of love, is always the great healer.

6) Remember, whatever you put out to another will come back to you. If you want hate, be hateful; if you want love, be love. If you want sensitive, deep, and meaningful sex, be sensitive and deep yourself. If you want a passionate and sexy lover, be passionate and sexy yourself. If you want to find a soul mate, be in soui communion with yourself and others.

7) Role swapping can be very beneficial to a love union. Make an appointment for this. The man dresses in women's clothes, the sexier the better, and the woman dresses in men's clothes. Put on some sensual music and meet as if you are at a club. Stay in your swapped roles as you get to know each other. Flirt and dance together, and finally do a slow sensual strip-tease for each other. If you wish, stay in the role reversal while making love afterward. You may learn a lot from this experience.

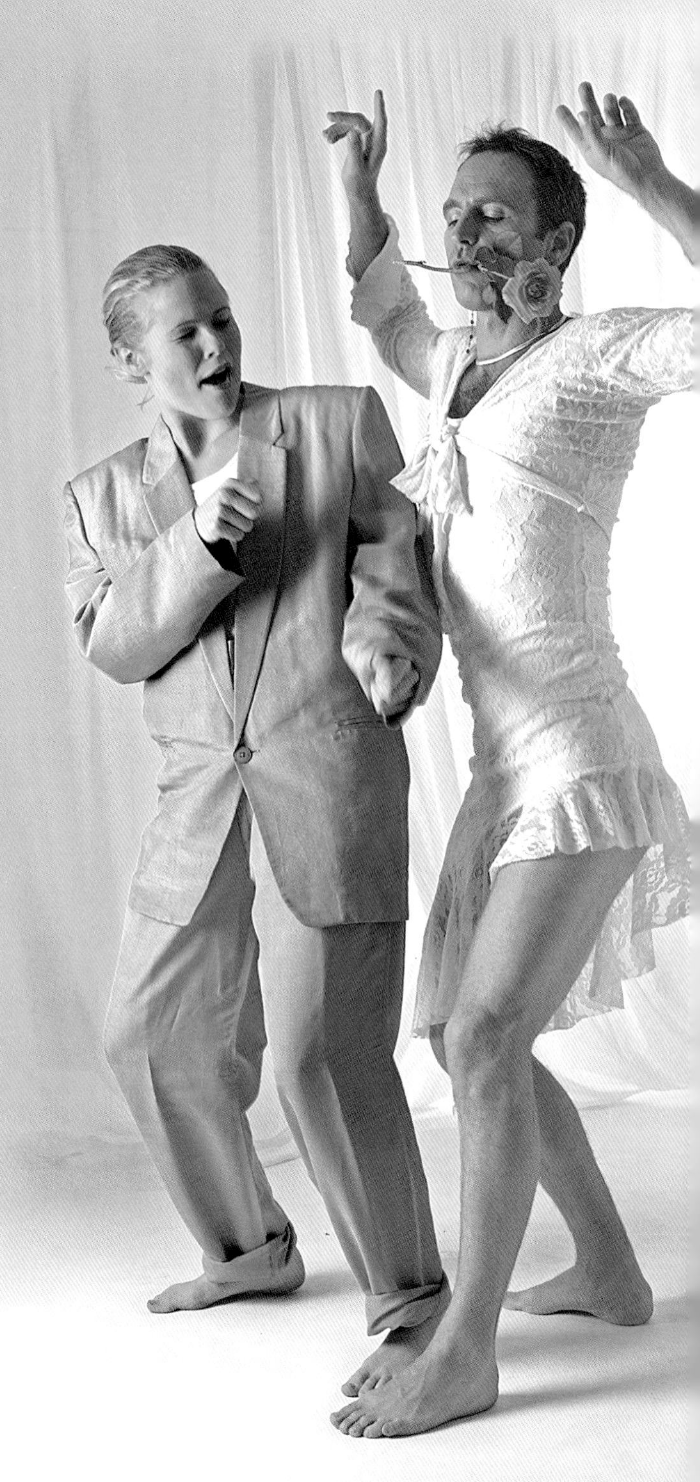

8) All these tips on communication can be applied to sexual union. Many people feel frustrated about their sex life but do not know how to change it. Clear, non-judgemental communication of your truth, from the heart, while using Yin vision, will do wonders. Do not be afraid to say what you need, and fully expect to give it to yourself first. Do you want to be touched just so on your clitoris? Be the first one to do it. If you are without inhibition about it, your partner will soon catch on. Would you like to enter a fully ready wet and juicy Yoni and move into full-body orgasm, while your partner praises god that you exist? Then learn how to be vibrant and orgasmic in your whole body and you will certainly discover this in a partner.

9) Your fantasies arise from different aspects of yourself, and are trying to teach you something. By understanding them rather than repressing them, you can be transformed.

♡ Fantasies from a repressed aspect of the self arise from inhibitions or conditioning. Many people do not allow themselves to enjoy their raw sexual impulses in a natural way. The mind will then seek ways of expressing this unlived energy through thoughts and fantasies. Tantra helps to open the natural flow of energy, restoring a healthy and fulfilling sexuality.

♡ Fantasies from an unlived aspect of the self arise from stagnation in the energetic system that has its origin in childhood. For example, sadomasochistic fantasies may stem from childhood experiences of physical punishment, which may create the imprint that "love" is expressed in this way. Fantasies such as rape, sexual domination, urinating or defecating on a partner, are all symptoms of childhood traumas. These traumas can be healed through childhood healing work, such as psychotherapy, regression therapy, family constellation therapy, color light therapy, and hypnosis.

♡ Fantasies from an instinctual source are natural fantasies that arise from our animal nature, such as threesomes. Fantasies around making love in different positions, oral sex, and others of this kind are very natural and can be played with. You do not actually have to live the fantasy – acting it out as a play will fulfil it and free you. However, if your fantasy will not harm another or yourself, and your partner is willing to enter into it, then it can be fun to do it with self-acceptance and playfulness. You could devote one love session to his fantasy, and another to hers. The partner in the supporting role should act the part he or she is assigned during the entire love session.

♡ Fantasies also arise from the soul level. The soul carries a desire to create a bridge of communication whereby the light of the spirit can become embodied, and orgasm is a door to a direct merging with soul and spirit. Fantasies from this level include: the longing to become one with a lover; the longing to become soul mates; the desire to be so fused that there is no question of separation or abandonment; the wish for your lover to know intuitively your deepest longings, secrets, and desires; the desire for a sexual union that continues forever; the desire to be in love on all levels, mentally, emotionally, physically, and spiritually.

The fantasy of discovering sacred sexuality and transcendent love is very healthy. It is, in essence, the longing for Tantra and spiritual awakening through sensuality.

10) Remember that the love that you experience, both the highs and the lows, is not dependant upon the person who is currently the conduit of love. Love is omnipresent and your lover is simply an excuse for you to access it. Through him or her you can dive deep into an experience of your own potential for becoming one with the heartbeat of the universe. Just as a fish may not recognize the ocean because he is in it, so we may not recognize the ocean of love we live in. The lover is a reminder. And if this lover disappears from your life, it does not mean that love itself has disappeared. The steps you have taken deep into love's embrace are yours forever. Lovers come and go, love remains.

love magic for singles

Whatever happens in life is preceded first by imagination and then actualized through our intent. If you are looking for a partner, this exercise can bring about magical results.

♡ Make a list of all the attributes you would like to find in a lover – physical, emotional, mental, and spiritual. Remember to include in your list that this person loves and is attracted to you, and vice versa.

♡ Look at your list and make sure that you have not made contradictory requests.

♡ Now, make a list of all your own attributes.

♡ Compare the lists. Do you have the ingredients needed within yourself to match this "dream partner"? If not, you have some homework to do. Start manifesting in yourself the qualities that will complement your dream lover.

♡ After one month, check your lists again and see if they have become balanced. Make any changes you need to make on the lists so that they feel compatible.

♡ Place these lists in a special place in your house dedicated to love and be receptive for what you have proposed to manifest.

Remember that a little imperfection adds spiceto life. Learning to accept human frailties adds depths of understanding to love and brings compassion toward oneself and others.

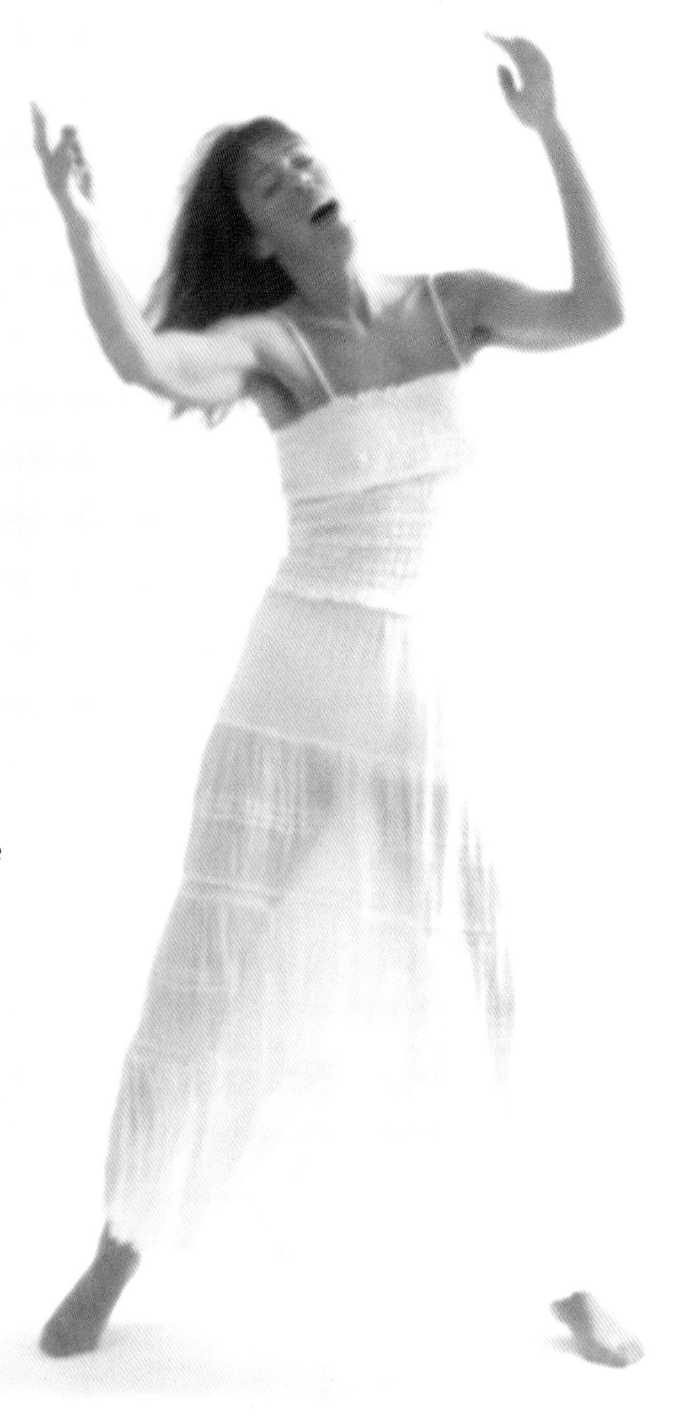

love magic for couples

This powerful exercise may take a day, a week, or even a month to complete. Follow your own rhythm, practicing the exercise in regular sittings, until you are ready for the sharing phase.

If your partner does the exercise as well, this will enhance its transforming power. However, it is important not to share what is on your lists until you have both reached the final step, since this will interfere with the process and make it harder to achieve a positive result. As you each have your own rhythm for the process, one partner may have to wait until the other is ready to begin the sharing.

♡ Make a list of everything you dislike about your partner – physically, emotionally, and mentally.

♡ In a column beside it, make a list of everything you love in your partner – physically, emotionally, and mentally.

♡ Compare the two lists. Which one is longer? Is there something you can delete from the dislike list? Is there anything you can add to the love list? Continue with this process, either in one or several sittings, until the love list is very long and the dislike list has only one or two key elements.

♡ At the same time, make the same lists about yourself. As you look at your own lists, look at your naked body in a mirror. This gives the experience more potency, since our bodies often reflect our likes and dislikes about ourselves.

During each sitting, try to cancel one or more qualities from the dislike list, and to add qualities to the love list. When the love list is very long, and the dislike list has perhaps one or two items on it, you are then ready to begin sharing with your partner.

sharing

♡ Write out the new lists you have developed through the exercise and burn the old ones. Then, get together with your lover and share from the heart. It is not necessary to tell your lover about all the things you had on the dislike list. Just stay with the lists as they are now. Let him or her know all the qualities that you love in him or her, and in yourself.

♡ Next, let your partner know that there are one or two elements you find difficult to love in yourself, and ask him or her for any suggestions on how to learn to dissolve these knots.

♡ Then, let your partner know there are one or two elements in him or her that you have difficulty accepting. Again, ask if he or she has any feelings on how these knots in your relating can be dissolved.

♡ By the end of this sharing you both may have found a creative way of moving through the obstacles in your love. Focusing on love is a magic way of helping love to grow. The more powerful the love, the easier it is to dissolve misunderstanding, wounds, and unconscious behavior patterns.

chapter 24

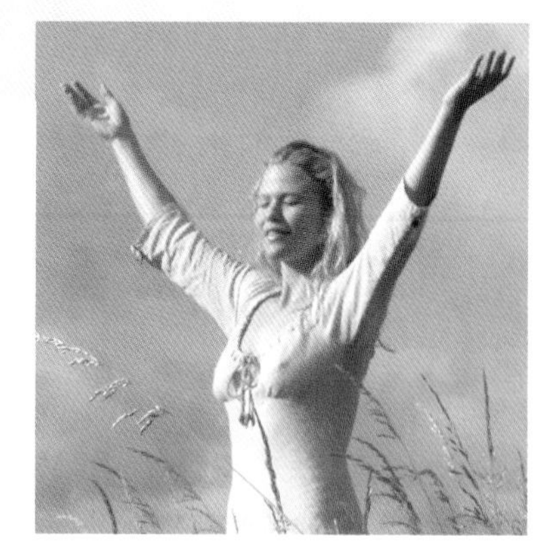

sensual, harmonious world

"By and by you see that a dance arises,
with the wind, with the sky, with the sun rays
coming through the trees, with the earth.
You are dancing.
You start feeling the pulse of the universe.
That is sexual.
Swimming in the river is sexual
Copulating is not the only sexual thing;
Anything where your body pulsates totally
With no inhibitions is sexual."
From *Zen, the Path of Paradox*, Osho

When you are flowing and alive in your sensuality, the whole world appears luminous and you have a smile on your lips for the people you meet. You are in a space of overflowing energy and delight. Perhaps you have had this experience: after a superb night of sex with a lover, the next day you feel as if you are floating on air. Your steps are buoyant, you feel abundant and generous, you want to kiss the world. The whole of nature appears to be sparkling and even mundane jobs become light and playful.

The fact that this happens proves that this state of being, this natural high, is part of the body's resources, to be accessed at any time. This "high" gets woken up by good sex, but is not dependent on sex in order to happen. Young children are on a natural high, in tune with existence and floating in a sea of love. Animals are also in this state. When you look into the eyes of a cat or dog you may see joy or peace, which awakens the same quality in you. Pets can teach us how to enter into a relaxed and easy state of being.

A love affair with life

You can learn how to awaken your dormant sensual aliveness so that it becomes a constant bubbling up of joy and fulfilment. You can become orgasmic and in love with life on an ongoing basis. To activate this, allow yourself to be really sensual. Let orgasmic energy spread all over your body, and into your actions, however mundane. When watering the garden, become one with it: dance with the trees swaying in the breeze; become the warmth of the sun kissing the flowers; become the bee, drinking nectar; become the butterfly; savor the smell of the rich earth; fall in tune with all of nature and dance with it.

When sitting silently anywhere, whether on a beach or on a bus, bring awareness to your breath. Let your breath activate pleasure all over your body. In a natural, flowing state the simple act of breathing creates a constant, pleasurable, inner massage. Breath is life, and it contains within it all the secrets of how to be fully vibrant and ecstatic.

We were born to dance. The body loves joyous exercise: some body functions, such as lymph flow, need physical activity to activate them. The best forms of exercise are those that bring a lot of pleasure, such as walking in nature, swimming in the sea, dancing, etc. Free-form dance is an easily accessible way to free inhibitions, open the flow of vital energy, and enter into inner ecstasy. Give yourself the gift of joyous exercise and you will soon find that you are naturally orgasmic a great deal of the time. Whenever Sarita's 84-year-old mother feels any ache or pain, she puts on some dance music, dances with abandon for 20 minutes, and all discomfort passes. She has discovered an ancient secret of health and longevity, which dancing cultures such as those in Brazil or Africa have known for a long time.

Ecstasy in everyday life

Touch is an essential ingredient in the awakening of sensual pleasure. How you treat your skin has a great impact on how you experience the world, and hugging and cuddling are the best ways to activate pleasure and wellbeing. The art of hugging is to feel and be present with the person you are with. Breathe together for a few moments, allowing your whole body to be in contact with the other person. Some people may be afraid of hugging because in many cultures it has sexual connotations. However, it is a very natural and deeply needed expression in all phases of life.

The quality contained in orgasm, which is an ecstatic let go into a space beyond time and mind, can be applied to everyday

In Holland there is an accredited university devoted to personal development, called the Humaniversity. They organize what they call "Social Meditations". In one of these, people gather in a public square and learn how to give perfect strangers a really good hug. You can imagine the scene, a big city square, full of people learning how to be present and loving with others through embrace.

life. When you laugh a great belly laugh, it has an orgasmic quality in it. This totality of expression can be brought into many areas: try drinking a cup of tea in an orgasmic way; dance naked under the full moon, making love with the moon and stars. Experiment with bringing that quality of celebrative and total let go into all areas of your life and discover how the world mirrors it back to you. For it is how you as an individual are inside, that is reflected back to you from the outside.

Creating harmony in society

A survey done in New York found that a certain area, normally prone to violence, became violence free at certain precise times on certain days in a seemingly inexplicable pattern. When further research was done into this phenomenon, the cause of the drop in violence was traced to a certain bus driver who covered that route. His demeanour was so overflowing with love and joy that it affected people all along his route, causing them to become more considerate of others. The reverse also happens. It has been found, when a boxing match is shown on TV, the next day levels of violence rise.

Many people carry the dream of a better world, where caring and easy joy are the norm. We may hope that this will come about through outward change of society as a whole, but this hope is an illusion. Society is made up of individuals and can only change through transformation of the individual. Thus we need to begin by transforming ourselves. If we are overflowing with sensuous and joyous aliveness, the people around us will benefit. In this way, one seed makes the whole earth green.

When we went to India to find our Tantra Master, we were searching for the essence of life. In time, having healed ourselves and found bliss, this energy began overflowing into offering individual sessions. Gradually, as we discovered the secret of bliss within relationships, the energy began overflowing into sharing through Tantra groups. And now this overflowing joy is being expressed through writing books. As people are touched by our energy, their own longing for personal transformation is ignited, and they begin the journey. One day, they also will begin overflowing and touching others.

The raising of personal consciousness, sensual fulfilment, and love are key ingredients for a harmonious and loving society. When a single heart is ignited by love, this moves like wildfire to other hearts, creating a pool of love in the collective unconscious. This pool inspires people everywhere to awaken to their inner potential for fulfilment, love, and consciousness. Good can be defined as that which happens in a state of expanded consciousness, leading to heightened sensitivity. The two examples in the box (left) illustrate how sensitive the collective unconscious is to the vibrations emitted by others. Who you are creates the world.

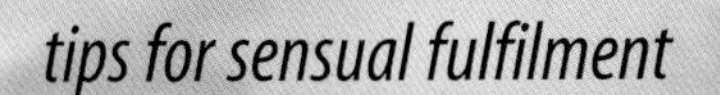

tips for sensual fulfilment

♡ Use every opportunity to revive your senses, so that you see, hear, taste, smell, and feel with heightened awareness, amplifying the pleasure of these experiences.

♡ Bring awareness to your breath. Feel your belly rising and falling. Allow the breath to massage your body from the inside, awakening pleasure and emotional aliveness.

♡ Move into regular joyous exercise, such as dancing, walking in nature, or swimming.

♡ Let living in community with others become communion. Express love through physical contact; touch and hug more.

♡ Become orgasmic in many facets of your life, in song, laughter, tears, and in nature. Let yourself have a love affair with life.

♡ Remember that you are creating the world each moment through your speech and actions and simply through who you are.

chapter 25

marriage of love and meditation

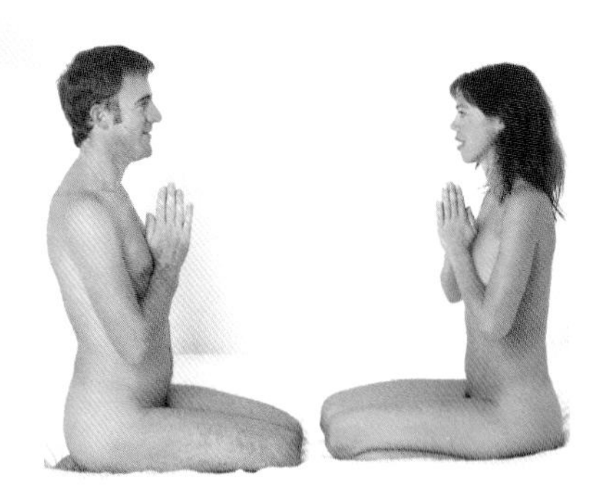

"Here in this body are the sacred rivers
Here are the sun and moon
As well as all the pilgrimage places
I have not encountered another temple
As blissful as my own body."
Saraha Doha, excerpt from Tantric scripture
translated by Nik Douglas

Tantra is a whole life approach that includes science, medicine, astrology, mathematics, music, art, architecture, worship, meditation, sexuality, and sensuality. It involves the practice of methods aimed toward personal transformation and spiritual awakening. There are two components of this transformative experience – meditation and love.

Meditation is a non-judgemental, witnessing consciousness. If you can become a non-judgemental observer of your own body, emotions, and mind you will be able to discover the refined aspect of these dimensions of your being. These refined aspects are divine, since each aspect of life is exalted, or of divine origin. When a meditator – a scientist of the inner world – attains to a state of pure awareness, he or she merges with that divine essence. This state has often been called enlightenment. The meditator realizes their oneness as a co-creator in the divine play of life. They become aware that the vibrations they emit affect the whole of creation and this knowledge awakens their sense of responsibility as a co-creator. The meditator becomes sensitive, with a keen and penetrating intelligence. The perfume of this state is love and compassion. The path of meditation is often chosen by men, as its scientific nature appeals to the male mind.

Women often choose the path of love, since the quality of heartfelt devotion is inherent in it. On this path there is usually an object of devotion to whom you surrender and by whose grace you are transformed. The object of devotion can be considered like a waterfall of higher consciousness, which pours itself into the receptive heart of the devotee. The feelings that well up in the devotee transport him or her to higher planes of awareness and consciousness. The overwhelming love that arises in the devotee is like a fire, burning away all that is impure, leaving only a pure flame of consciousness.

This transcendental love is the refined aspect of what we call love. In normal love, passion and many emotions are present. In transcendental love, ordinary love is transformed to its exalted aspect through total surrender to a higher consciousness. The devotee comes to know and understand that the whole universe is made only of love – all else is illusion. This understanding gives rise to inner ecstasy, compassion, heightened sensitivity, and intelligence. The devotee knows the whole of life as a divine manifestation. The perfume of such realization is gratefulness.

Reclaiming your potential

Practiced alone, the path of meditation may be dry; it has a resonance with scientific enquiry. The path of love, if practiced alone, tends to be ungrounded and imbued with hallucination; it is in tune with the artistic temperament. Just like man and woman, these two paths are opposite and yet complementary aspects of one truth. In the lineage of Tantra we practice, these two paths are fused. The symbol of this fusion, and the object of veneration in Tantra temples, is a sculpted Lingam resting within a sculpted Yoni. The Lingam represents godliness in its male aspect and the Yoni represents godliness in its female aspect. The teaching is clear: male and female genitals are made as complementary opposites, both necessary for creation to manifest. This simple logic can also be applied to the spiritual path. Wherever there are two opposites, when they are joined as complementary aspects of one whole, there in that meeting of opposites we discover the ultimate truth.

This same simple key can be used to unlock all the secrets of the universe. In Tantra, the human being is seen as a microcosm mirroring the macrocosm. Therefore Tantric meditation uses the body and its functions as the object of meditation – a jumping board into universal consciousness. Tantra includes everything in the body or mind in this scientific research. All aspects of the human experience are considered worthy of attention. When this attitude is joined with the feminine, heart-oriented, devotional

"The meditations have opened me to experience my deepest longings, to know my roots as a woman, and to find deep connection to earth, mother earth. I feel that deep connection in lovemaking in ways I have never experienced before, becoming earth, and opening, surrendering to the universe. This has opened me to my partner in ways I have never known before, experiencing the energy of man and woman in truth. We have a wonderful deep connection of love I didn't know possible, that was only a dream before."

Rachel, Tantra group participant

approach, each aspect of life is considered divine. The body is viewed as a temple; the act of love between a man and a woman is sacred and held in the highest esteem, as an opportunity to embrace the most exalted spiritual states. The man and woman, opposite and yet complementary, become teachers for one another, for in the understanding and union of the two, awakened consciousness can be found.

Every lover, deep down, senses this potential in the act of love. This is why so many people hope to discover perfect love, and why they despair when they cannot find it. It is an essential human longing to know God through human love. When we see people moving into the Tantra experience for the first time, they generally exclaim, "I always knew this was possible. It is what I have dreamed of for a long time! I just didn't know how to access it." They feel like this because Tantra is a remembrance arising from the inside. This remembrance is of your very nature and is a reclaiming of your potential.

"Tantra meditation created a space for me to let go into myself and take playfully those things that prevented me from letting go into infinite love and my spark of light. It taught me to connect with myself and my soul-mate, creating that 'coming home' feeling."

Sally, Tantra group participant

Practicing Tantra methods

Since Tantra revolves around method, its path can only fully be understood by those who practice the methods, and by doing so, are transformed. This is why, traditionally, Tantra has been passed on as a personal transmission from Master to disciple.

The meditations and exercises in this book help to anchor the meeting of love and meditation through Tantra practice. To enter into these, first consecrate the space. Bring a loving awareness to it – this may include cleaning it, decorating it with special cloth, perhaps using flowers, incense, and candles. Then invite higher consciousness to be present to support you in the method.

Another way of supporting your entry into Tantric meditation is to make appointments for your practice, and then to honour these appointments no matter what. This simple device will enable you to place your Tantra practice in a position of priority in your life. Tantric meditations can take from a few minutes to one hour, depending on the method, so they can be fitted into the busiest lifestyle.

For CDs with guided Tantra meditations, see the Resources section, page 188.

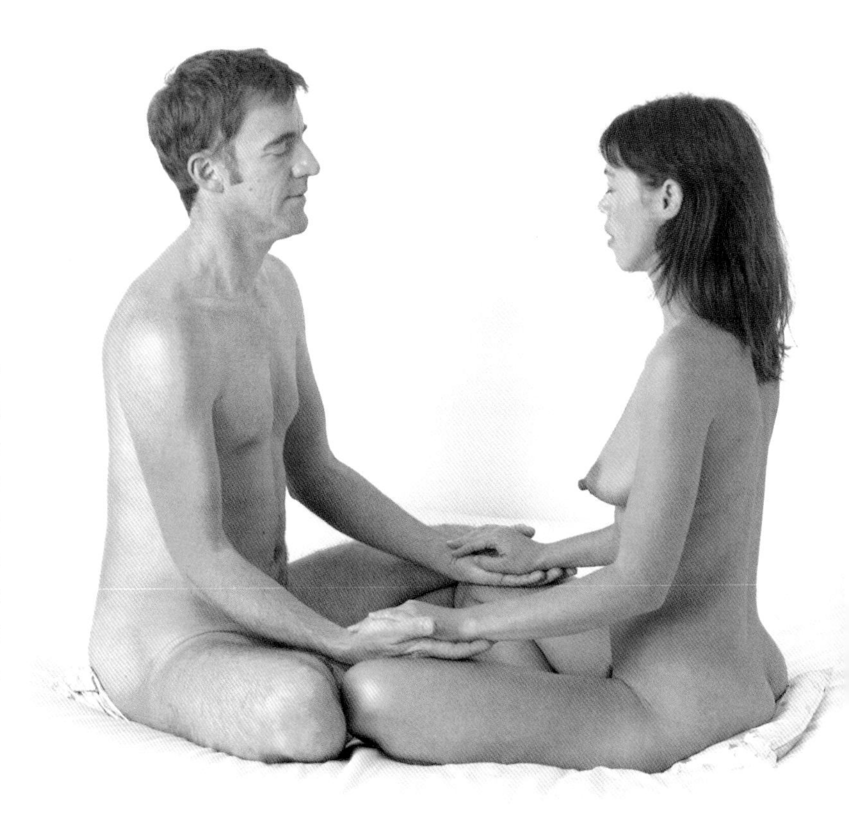

bio-resonance

This Tantra meditation can be practiced with a lover, to bring resonance and harmony to the male–female dynamic.

♡ **Phase 1:** (10 minutes) Sit opposite your partner, with your palms touching and fingers resting lightly on your partner's wrists. With your eyes closed, and breathing normally, simply witness your breathing, your mind, and your emotions as an impartial observer. This position automatically creates harmony in the bio-electricity within your own body, and between you and your partner.

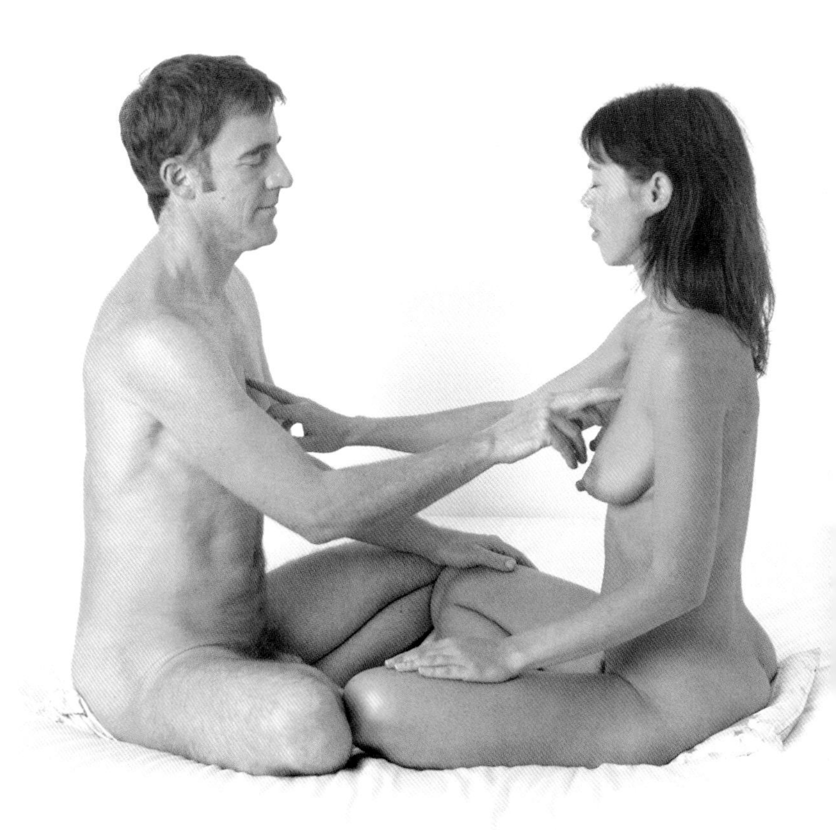

♡ **Phase 2:** (3 minutes) Simultaneously, each place the middle finger of your right hand on your partner's heart chakra, in the center of the chest. This creates a heart resonance between you.

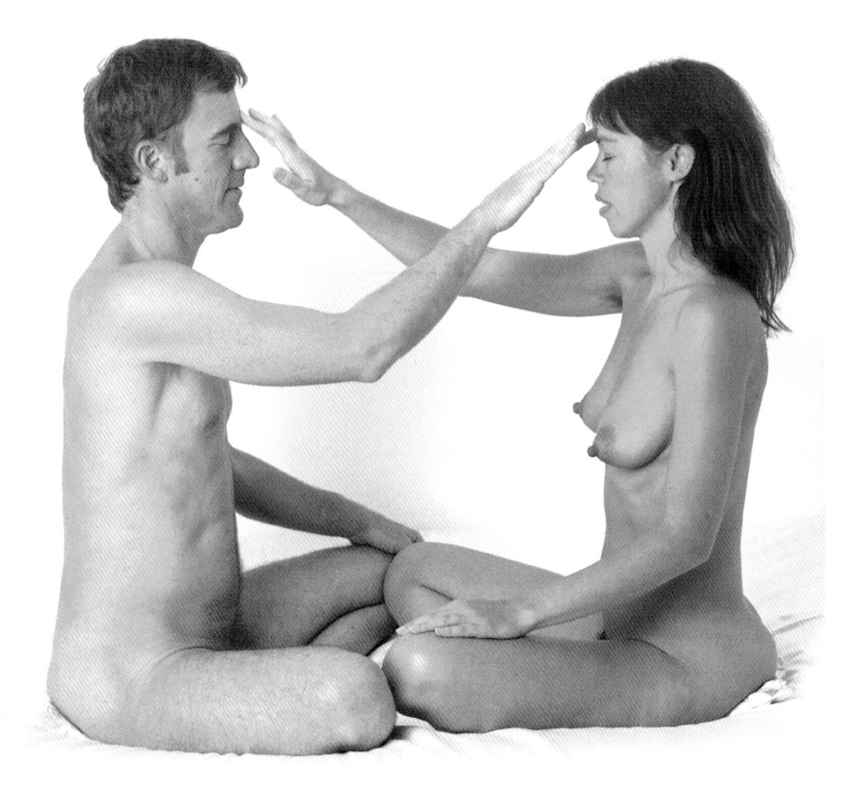

♡ **Phase 3:** (3 minutes) Simultaneously, each place the middle finger of your right hand on your partner's third eye center, between the eyebrows. This will create a resonance in your intuition.

♡ **Phase 4:** (10 minutes) With your palms touching and fingers resting lightly on your partner's wrists, create resonance of the voice by humming together. Humming activates the crown chakra and the central channel, bringing an awakening of spiritual energy.

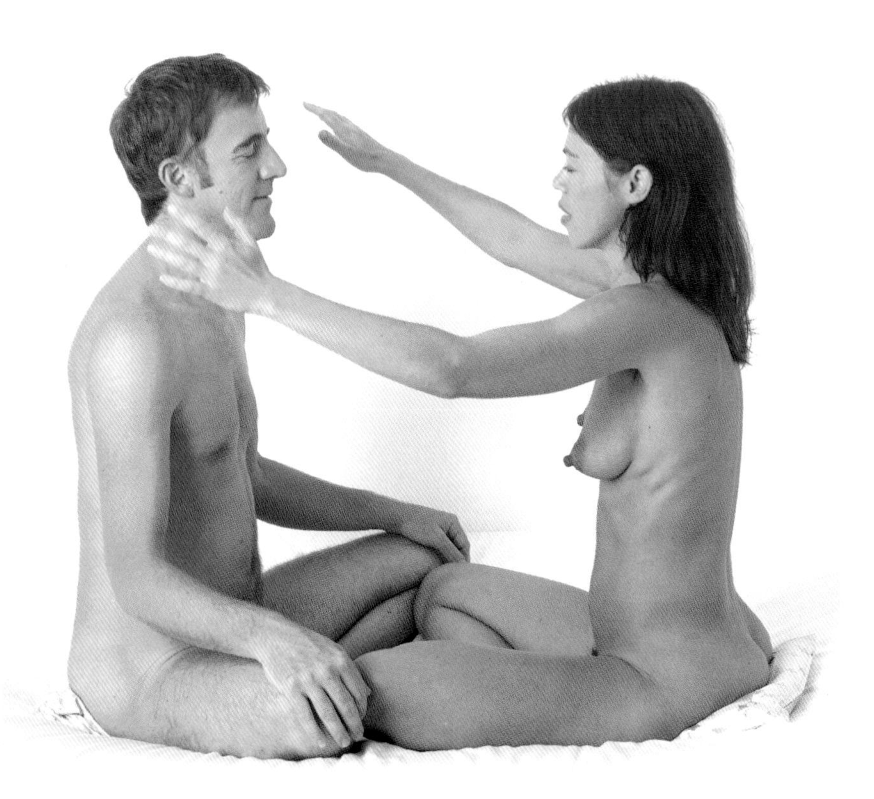

♡ **Phase 5:** (10 minutes) Take turns to touch the whole of your partner's body, wherever you can reach. The touch is loving and firm, anchoring the resonance in the physical body. Then caress your partner's aura with your hands, around the physical body. The receiving partner sits with eyes closed and in silence throughout.

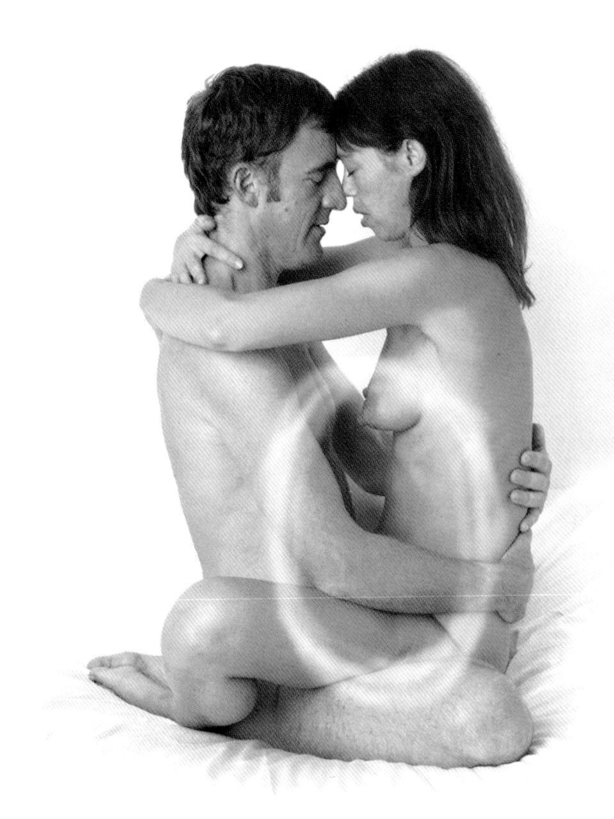

♡ **Phase 6:** (10 minutes) You can both have your eyes open or closed for this stage. Either remain seated opposite each other or move into the Yab Yum position, with the Lingam inside the Yoni or not as you wish. If the Lingam is inside the Yoni, you are not moving toward genital release, but simply relaxing together in the state called "plugging in" (see page 109).

Now enter into a phase of circular breathing. For the first 5 minutes the man breathes out through his Lingam. As he does so, the woman inhales the breath through her Yoni, raises the breath upward, and breathes out through her heart. As she does so, the man breathes in through his heart, allows the breath to descend, and breathes out through his Lingam, and so on. If you wish, one of you can show the breathing circle through hand gestures.

For the next 5 minutes, reverse the breathing circle. The woman breathes out through her Yoni as the man breathes in through his Lingam. He raises the breath, and then breathes out through his heart. As he does so, the woman breathes in through her heart, allows the breath to descend, and then breathes out through her Yoni, and so on. This phase activates the main positive poles in both partners and also helps to awaken their inner male and inner female aspects so that the experience of transformation through Tantra can flower.

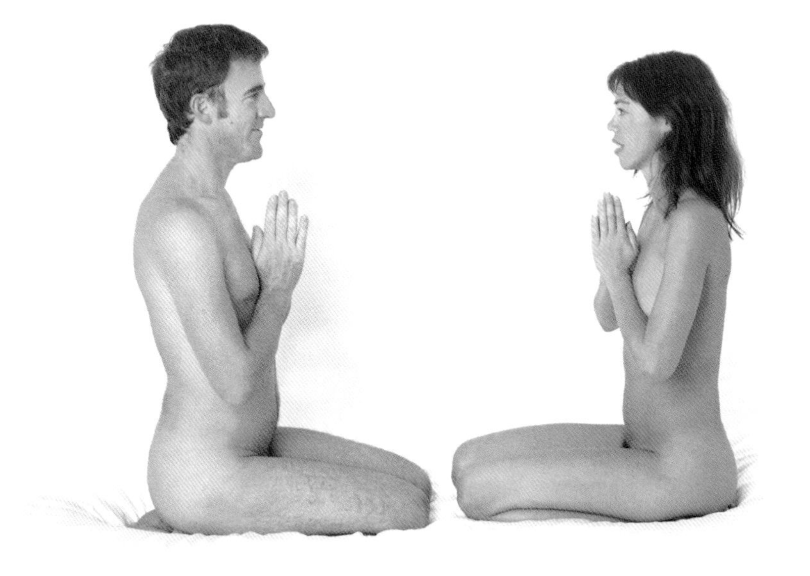

♡ **Phase 7:** Namaste, looking into each other's eyes (see page 100), and then bow down, crown chakras touching, to express your gratitude for this shared meditation.

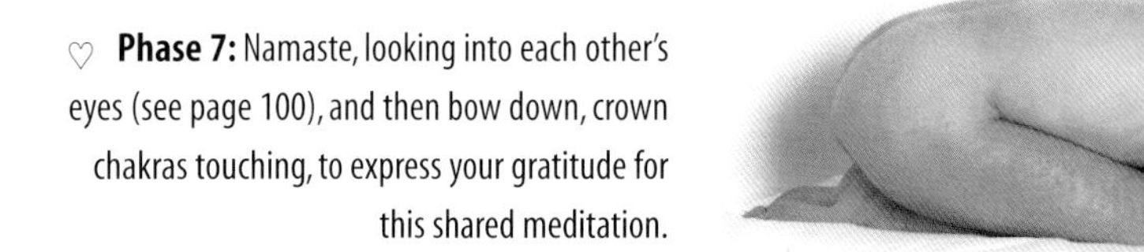

chapter 26

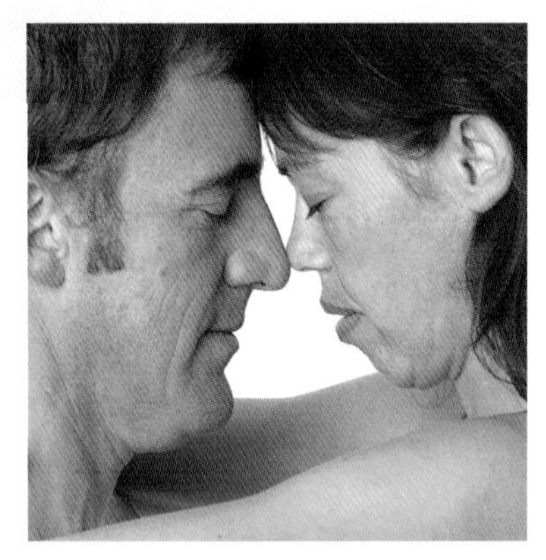

from sex to superconsciousness

"Space is the Lingam, the earth is its Yoni.
Within it dwell all the Gods."
Skanda Purana, ancient Indian chronicle

The journey from sex to superconsciousness is one of the beautiful contributions Tantra offers to the world. Human beings have only one energy, and in its raw, unrefined state this is sex. Through the practice of Tantra, your sexual energy becomes refined, leading you on a path into spiritual awakening. Superconsciousness is the flower that arises from a sexuality lived with the intelligence of Tantra.

In India, the lotus has long been the symbol of spiritual awakening. Sex is like the mud from which the glorious lotus flower arises – without this mud there would be no lotus. This simple illustration encapsulates the whole vision of Tantra. A person on the Tantra path will greatly respect the raw energy of sex and at the same time will seek to refine this energy to its ultimate potential.

If you are cut off from your sexual energy you are also cut off from the potential for elevated consciousness, because you are an organic whole – your mind, body, and emotions function as one organism.

People are often afraid of their sexuality because it is linked with animality. They may think that through embracing their sexuality they will move into a sub-human state, where gross licentiousness leads into a downward spiral, ending in the loss of culture and refinement. In fact, the exact opposite is true. When sexuality is repressed it lurks in the subconscious of the body/mind, growing and expanding until finally it erupts into perversion of all kinds. Along the way it tortures the person who is involved in this repression, through dreams and fantasies.

When a whole culture subscribes to the idea of repressing sexuality, it creates an environment where violence, depression, and fanaticism flourish. Eventually the culture erupts into licentious, perverted, and pornographic behaviour. The danger is that since intelligence has not been applied to this type of sexual expression, it leads you into unconsciousness and despair. You cannot find a way of refining this energy and helping it to grow into a lotus flower of love and consciousness.

A tree that is prevented from growing straight will find a different way to grow, perhaps twisting around a rock. Each tree is programmed to seek the light, and it will do so, even if this means growing toward the light in a twisted and warped way. We carry the urge to move toward the light of higher consciousness. But this is only possible if you have an aware rootedness in sex, like a tree is rooted in the earth. If their natural growth patterns are prevented, humans will find warped ways of contacting their sexual energy, because they need it to survive, to grow, and to come to fruition.

Spiritual awakening

Tantra is a life approach that accepts people as they are. It simply applies the science of meditation to the human condition, to refine it to its ultimate potential. If you bring a meditative consciousness to the sex act, you will soon find that this act is transformed into love. And if you continue with this approach, sex and love are transformed into spirituality, a merging with the whole. In this way, sex itself becomes a divine experience. There is a saying in Tantra, that sex and Samadhi (spiritual awakening) are one. This realization comes to the Tantra practitioner.

If you bring a meditative consciousness to the sex act, you will soon find that this act is transformed into love. And if you continue with this approach, sex and love are transformed into spirituality, a merging with the whole. In this way, sex itself becomes a divine experience.

The Rudra Veena is an Indian musical instrument made with two big gourds, one at either end of a central spine. It is said to represent the human being, with the head at one end, the tail at the other, and the spine in the middle. The strings of the instrument lie along the spine and the musician plays the music of life between the two polarities, by activating the spine and allowing the resonance to travel between them. The music of the Rudra Veena is believed to come closest to the soundless sound, the sound of the ultimate, represented by the symbol "Aum". Of course, training is needed to play such sublime music. The discipline and dedication the musician brings to learning an instrument can also be applied to sex and relating. Then you discover the miracle of sex and Samadhi as two poles of one energy, finally merging one with the other.

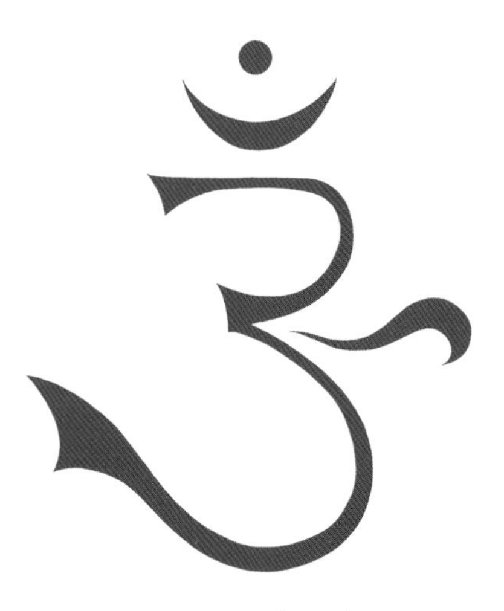

five steps from sex to superconsciousness

Following these five steps, using the techniques described in earlier chapters, allows your sexual energy to refine to its ultimate potential.

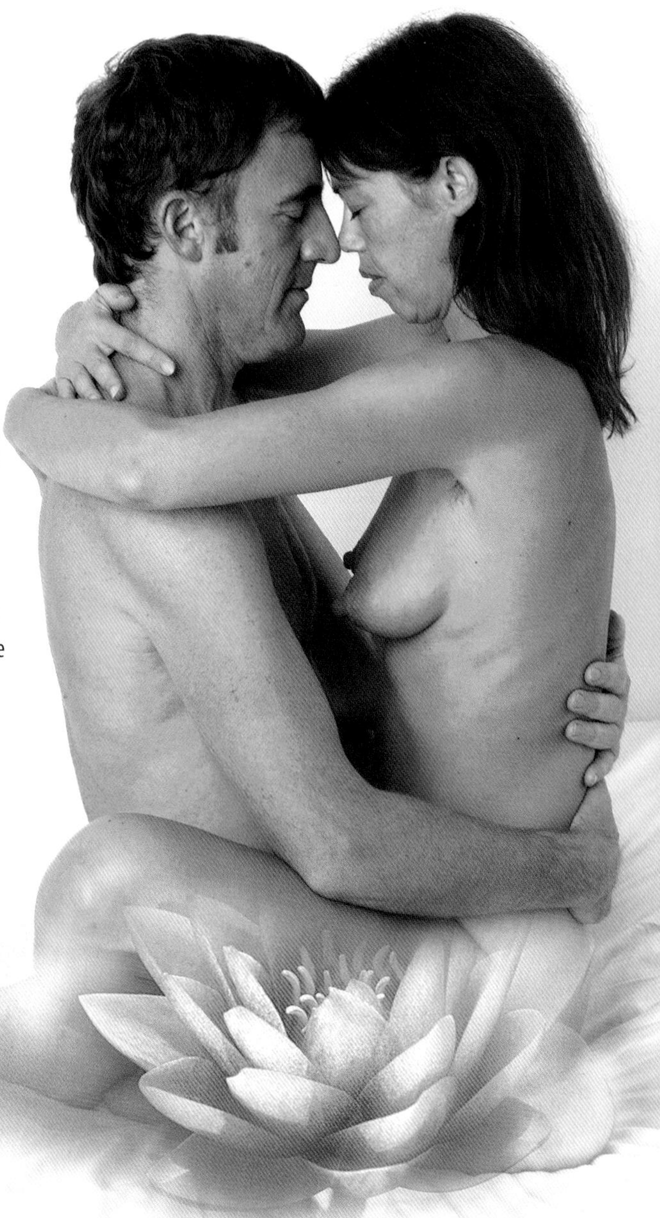

♡ Bring a meditative awareness to the sex act. This does not mean controlling it, but rather allowing sexuality to be expressed fully within the context of meditation and sacredness.

♡ Free trapped emotional energies. You need to be in contact with and express your emotions without psychologically harming or wounding another person.

♡ Develop extrasensory awareness. Awaken your senses so that the hidden sensitivity of each one begins to function. The awakening of the hidden senses is known as the opening of the third eye, the third ear, the second touch, the second smell and taste.

♡ The steps above lead to the awakening of genius. Becoming vast enough to contain the contradictions of life within yourself opens the door to wisdom. In that point of meeting you will discover truth and genius, which has a unique expression for each individual.

♡ The final step is awakened consciousness – the blossoming of a thousand-petalled lotus at the crown chakra. It is also known as the snake eating its own tail, or the source and the goal as one. This is where sex and Samadhi are known as one energy. In Tantra it is called Mahamudra, the great gesture that arises out of the cosmic orgasm. Now you will be able to embrace the whole. You will step from the known into the abyss beyond the mind, the unknown. You become simply an open channel for universal consciousness.

Jivan, a musician and management consultant, and Agyana, mother and personal development facilitator, have been together for 10 years. Their relationship was transformed by an experience of superconsciousness during lovemaking, following Tantra training.

Jivan: We were honoring the Lingam and Yoni simultaneously. We were moving slowly, not going for orgasm, just being present with each other.

Agyana: In the past, it would have been a mutual blow-job. This was different.

Jivan: We were one body. Her orgasm was my orgasm. It was tremendous joy, laughter.

Agyana: In the past, I have felt anxiety that he could go on to a greater level of excitement, leaving me behind. This time, I followed my feeling to stroke his perineum. It was incredibly powerful. I felt the vibration of the stimulation I was giving to him in my clitoris and my third eye.

Jivan: We were one. What was happening in her happened in me, and vice versa. Before, we have had moments of extreme closeness. But this time the thin veil that separates us was gone.

Agyana: The first level of intimacy could be called simultaneous pleasure. This experience we are describing crosses over from separate but simultaneous to us becoming one body. The experience is that of sun and moon meeting, the warmth in moonlight and cool beauty in sunlight, Yin and Yang merged as one.

Since that experience, there is a feeling that all the busy-ness of life doesn't touch our unity. Something has remained, even when we are challenged by childcare, or work. There is a deeper quality of togetherness, which remains untouched by outward events. This brings a deep trust and security in our relationship. The depth of connection we have has swept away the insecurity that I used to feel, such as the concern that he could have an affair. The depth we have is so total that anything else would simply be a ripple on the surface.

Jivan: I feel much freer to be as I am, mischievous, flirtatious, or whatever. I feel free, and yet more in touch with the love, the depth, of connection I have with her. I would like to say to lovers everywhere, keep going. Don't stop half way. Go on until you either separate or transform. Feel honestly and be really honest with yourself. Let go of the voices that prevent you from being really close and intimate. Dare to be vulnerable. Ask for a hug. Get into her lap. Let her cuddle you. Allow your little boy to emerge and discover God in the process. It is not until you get real that you can walk together to the promised land.

Agyana: My message to lovers everywhere is: keep going into the vulnerability. Keep showing your own vulnerability and calling for the vulnerability of your partner. The magic comes out of that space. It may be the scariest place, but it is where the magic is. Maybe there are layers of healing before the ecstasy can come. But it is really a deep pleasure when truths are revealed. The peak pleasure comes only after relaxing into the valley of exposing your ordinary truth.

chapter 27

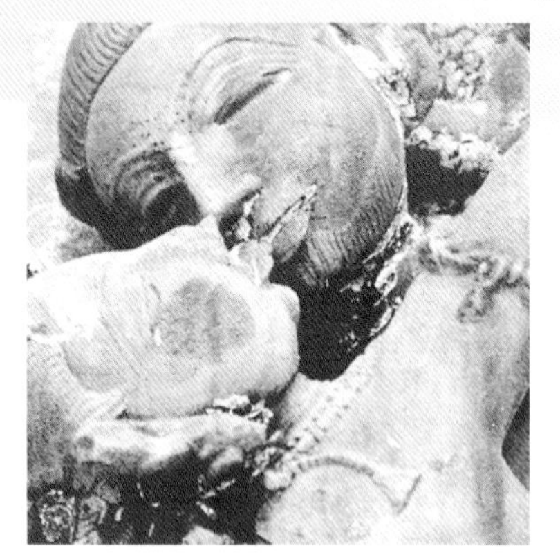

the wisdom of the ancients

"Sex contains all, bodies, souls,
Meanings, proofs, purities, delicacies, results, promulgations,
Songs, commands, health, pride, the maternal mystery, the seminal milk
All hopes, benedictions, bestowals,
All the passions, loves, beauties, delights of the earth,
These are contained in sex as parts of itself
And justifications of itself."
From *Poem of Procreation* (1856)Walt Whitman

Tantra arose deep in Indian pre-history, from the merging of two distinct religious approaches. One claimed the supreme origin of life to be female (Shakti), the other masculine (Shiva); both celebrated the sacred within the mundane, the body as a microcosm of the macrocosm. The Shivaistic approach had its roots in the Assours civilization, over 60,000 years ago. According to the Shiva *Puranas*, the Assours were masters of sun technology, and had three great cities, one of them in the sky. The roots of Shakti can be traced to the mother goddess, and fertility rites practiced by ancient peoples throughout the world. The symbol that expresses this merging is Ardhanareshvara, a deity who is half man, half woman.

Shiva and his consort Devi were in their house making love. Two gods, Brahma and Vishnu came to see Shiva for some important matter. When they saw he was making love, they politely waited outside. However, he was so involved in the adoration of his beloved that they waited six hours, and still he showed no signs of stopping his rapturous embrace. They became angry and cursed him, saying that from now on he would only be known through his genitals. This is why the inner sanctum of Shiva temples holds a carved stone phallus, the Shiva Lingam, resting in a carved Yoni.

Tantric sages understood that the essence of life is in the meeting of opposite yet complementary polarities. They believed that the sun, moon, stars, oceans, rivers, mountains – everything existing in the heavens and on earth – are represented within the human body. From this understanding they developed a cosmology through the sensitive worship and scientific analysis of male and female bodies, focusing particularly on the secrets of birth, death, and immortality encoded in sex. Tantric cosmology is based solely on deep introspective research, through powerful consciousness-raising methods. Anyone who attained superconsciousness through the practice of these methods was regarded as an incarnation of Shiva or Shakti, and a spiritual master.

Recognizing the presence of Shiva or Shakti in your partner can raise an ordinary sexual meeting into a truly divine and sacred experience. To facilitate this, Tantra sexual practices are surrounded by ritual and practiced in the context of meditation. These methods and rituals were taught by Gurus, who had through the practice of meditation reached expanded consciousness and, having attained inner wisdom, could offer a direct living transmission of Tantra to aspirants. One of the most famous of Tantra Masters, known as an incarnation of Shiva, gave to the world 112 methods of meditation for the attainment of expanded consciousness. Many of these use awakening of the senses as a door into refined consciousness, and some use lovemaking as meditation.

Tantra society was founded on the principle of attaining elevated consciousness through the practice of meditation in concert with love. This gave rise to magnificent architecture, great works of art, exquisite music, and a prosperous life-affirming culture. The most recent Tantra renaissance was from the time of Christ until the Mohammedan invasion of India, around 1100 AD. Some of the many Tantra temples constructed in India during this period can still be seen today. The most-well known, in Khajuraho, are renowned for their exquisitely carved statues, on the exterior walls, of people in every kind of sexual posture.

In western culture, worshipping the sex act, or revering the genitals in a temple seems completely alien. But it is based on a profound intelligence, with tremendous implications. If godliness is in the genitals, this makes spiritual principles easily accessible to human beings. It means that when you are making love, you are in contact with the divine. Thus the love act is something to be treated with the utmost respect, as the container for all that is most holy and exalted. Every lovemaking session can be considered an act of prayer.

"The highest of all values is love, and its fountain is in our body. The worship must start with the body of man. In the mortal frame resides the immortal."

From *Impact of Tantra on Religion and Art* by T N Mishra

The dawning of a new age

The ancient Indian chronicles known as the *Puranas* describe the cycles of creation. These cycles are divided into Yugas, or ages, which resemble the four legs of a table. During the first, golden age (Krita) the table has four legs, so the foundation of human society is solid and unwavering, firmly standing in truth, wisdom, love, and creativity. This phase lasts 24,195 years. During the second Yuga (Treta) the table has only three legs. Rules of

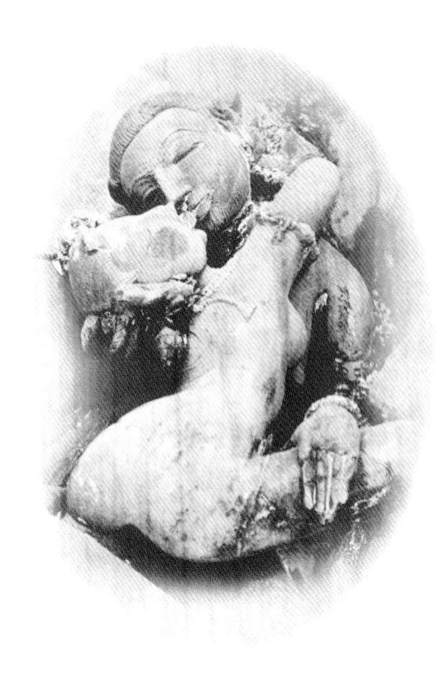

"A new man is striving to be born, a new consciousness is knocking on the doors. And the future is going to be that of Tantra, because now no more dual attitudes can hold man's mind."

Osho, contemporary Tantra master

conduct and ritual need to be established in order to keep the balance. Treta lasts 18,146 years. In the third Yuga (Dvapara), the table has only two legs. This is the age of doubt and instability, which lasts 12,097 years. In the fourth Yuga (Kali) the age of ignorance and conflict, the table has only one leg – it wobbles, all is chaos, and war is prevalent. This age lasts 6,048 years. Civilization crumbles, eventually giving way to a new golden age, where the first cycle of creation begins afresh. The first cycle of creation goes hand in hand with a Tantric approach to life.

At present we are in the sunset of the Kali Yuga, the age of ignorance, which began 3,606 years before Christ. The sunset of this Kali Yuga began in 1939 and is due to end in 2442 AD. During this age of chaos, human beings have a great opportunity to awaken spiritually because cosmic forces are accelerated. Similarly, the process of de-creation and ignorance is accelerated. Each of us has a choice: to take the downward spiral into mass destruction or to ride the ascending spiral into the new dawn. If the majority of people cling to the ignorance and violence inherent in the Kali Yuga, there will be cataclysmic destruction on a grand scale. In the sunset of the Kali Yuga, we can also sense the first subtle hints of the qualities of the new dawn. An ancient scripture, the *Kaula Tantra*, predicts that: "There is a brotherhood of Tantrics waiting to be brought to life. This brotherhood will awaken as the end of the Kali Age approaches. Recognizing the potent female principle of life, the brotherhood of Tantra will transform this polluted world. Then, at the ecstatic moment when one age transforms into the next, those faithful followers of the selfless path will reach their goal."

As time goes by, more people will come to understand the true importance of Tantra as a natural and refined approach to life, love, and spirituality. Since only a deeply fulfilled human being can be free, true freedom will only be possible when godliness again finds a home in the genitals. Fulfilment comes when sex and spirit are joined in a harmonious dance of life. Tantra offers the keys for every man and woman to know the celebration of sex and spirit within themselves. The healing of the separation of sex and spirit within each individual is also the healing of male–female dynamics and of society as a whole.

We are not saying that we have to go back to a so-called golden age to create a golden future. The natural law of life moves from order, to chaos, to a higher level of order. In this way, higher levels of evolution become possible. If we can embrace the evolutionary shift we are now in, embrace the chaos and learn from it, our learning curve will propel us into a completely new evolutionary step, which transcends all previous societies in its attainment of truth, wisdom, love, and creativity.

A vital aspect in this scenario is how to nurture the harmonious meeting of male and female energies. Within each one of us is carried the power and the possibility for this new dawn to become a reality through a sexuality lived with the intelligence of Tantra. The beauty of this approach is that we can discover wisdom through pleasure, through an intimate sensorial celebration of all that life is. Each time you enter into caring, conscious, ecstatic sex, you are in tune with the new dawn of humanity. You are in tune with the renewal of all of life.

"When my beloved returns to the house,

I shall make my body into a Temple of gladness

Offering this body as an altar of joy

My let-down hair will sweep it clean

Then my beloved will consecrate this temple."

Song from the Baul Mystics of India

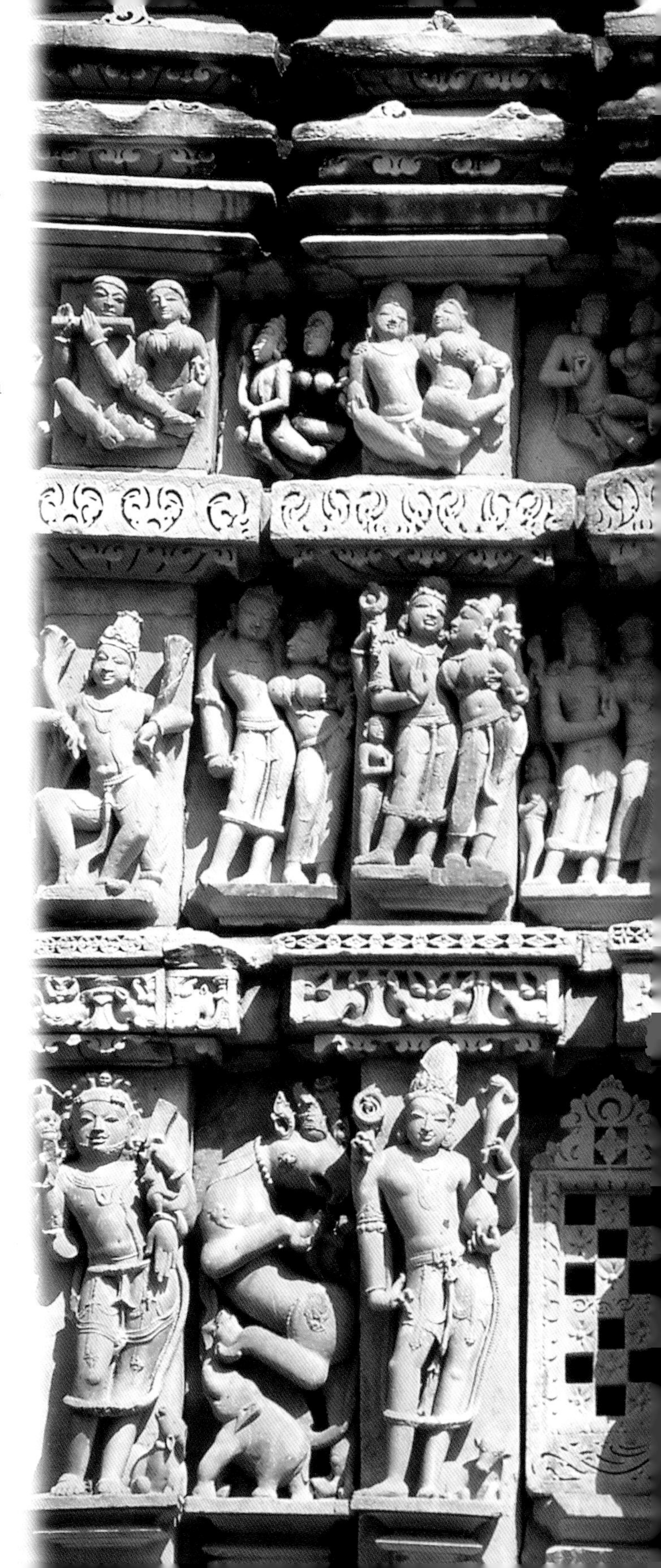

Menu of exercises

Use this "menu" to choose the most appropriate exercise or meditation for a particular time.

Exploring the peaks and valleys of love page 117 (For lovers) Making love in Yin and Yang holds the master key to fulfilling sex. This can revolutionize a couple's sex life. It is helpful in conservation of semen and to restore libido, and also for sexual dysfunction.

Enhance your love session page 123 Atmosphere and attitude can make all the difference for a fulfilling sexual experience. Try these secrets for heightened erotic pleasure.

Intelligent refinement of sex page 125 Helpful hints for nurturing a positive sexual relationship.

Children's meditation page 132 To be practiced with an adult carer. Children have so much energy and adults do not always know how to handle it. This meditation, designed especially for children, helps to channel a child's energy into a very positive direction, bringing harmony to the classroom or to family life.

Sex tips for girls page 136, **Sex tips for boys** page 137 Entering into the world of sexual expression as an adolescent can be a confusing, challenging, or difficult passage. These tips for boys and girls bring valuable clarity and understanding, supporting the adolescent in making intelligent sexual relating and lifestyle choices.

Tips for connecting with your lover page 141 Good for all lovers, and especially recommended for young adults. Valuable tips on taking time to tune into each other before and during lovemaking.

Embracing meditation page 146 Good for all lovers, and especially recommended for middle-aged couples. This is a valuable Tantra meditation to dissolve tension or discord, bring balance and harmony, and infuse sexual relations with the refined quality of conscious love. Helpful for "rising in love".

Keep attentive on the fire page 151 Good for all lovers, and especially recommended for elders. This Tantra meditation to be practiced during lovemaking helps you to discover the secret for retention of ejaculation, thereby supporting the possibility of continuing sexual pleasure as long as you live. It also helps to renew vigor, thereby supporting longevity, and supports a build-up of energy for spiritual development.

Caressing meditation page 157 (For lovers or friends) This Tantric meditation using touch is the original technique upon which some sex therapy is based. Enhances all-over body sensitivity, leading to heightened pleasure in sex. Especially nourishing for women. Helpful for all lovers and particularly recommended in the case of sexual dysfunction.

A meal you will never forget page 158 (Alone or with a lover) This sensorial Tantra meditation uses smell and taste, and is ideal as foreplay or after-play.

Looking with the eyes of love page 159 (Alone or with a lover) This Tantra meditation uses Yin vision to expand into deep love. It helps bring Yin and Yang aspects into balance and invites intimacy with your lover and the world around you.

Uncensored lovemaking page 160 (With a lover) This meditation uses sound, expression, and hearing to propel a couple into completely uninhibited expression during lovemaking. Cleanses repression, bringing freedom and intimacy.

Four-minute laughing meditation page 161 (Alone or with a lover) Laughter is beneficial to psychological and physical health. Similar to orgasm in its effect, it is a number one ingredient in a positive transformation of life energy.

Ten tips for deeper communication page 163 (For lovers) Tips to help you build deep and nourishing communication with your partner.

Love magic for singles page 166 If you are single but would like to find a lover who is just right for you, this technique can help.

Love magic for couples page 167 If you find discord arising between you and your partner, this method can help to dissolve its roots and to inspire a new chapter in your relationship, based on love and understanding.

Tips for sensual fulfilment page 171 (Alone) Sensual fulfilment can be an ongoing experience in each aspect of your life. Integrate these tips in your daily life and discover how vibrant and joyous you can become.

Bio-resonance page 175 (For lovers) This Tantra method brings harmonious resonance to the couple, using the bio-electricity of male/female opposite polarities, and working with sound, touch, and breath. It allows a refinement of sexual energy, deep intimacy, and oneness, and can lead to an experience of sacred sexuality and "rising in love".

Five steps from sex to superconsciousness page 180 These indicate how to access ultimate Tantra, called Mahamudra, the great gesture arising from orgasm with the universe. It is helpful for those who are interested in Tantra not only to enhance their sex lives, but also as a path to spiritual awakening.

Resources

Books

We have used the following books, listed by subject, in our research. We highly recommend these books as resources to help support a healthy sexual and spiritual lifestyle.

Sex and Tantra

Camphausen, Rufus C *The Yoni* Inner Traditions, 1996

Danielou, Alain *The Phallus* Inner Traditions, 1995
La Fantaisie des Dieux et L'aventure Humaine Rocher 1985

Douglas, Nik and Slinger, Penny *Sexual Secrets* Destiny Books, 2000

Hite, Shere *The New Hite Report* Hamlyn, 2000

Hsi Lai *The Sexual Teachings of the White Tigress* Destiny Books, 2001

Johari, Harish *Tools For Tantra* Destiny Books, 1986

Kaplan, Helen Singer *The New Sex Therapy: Active Treatment for Sexual Dysfunctions* Pelican, 1978

Khanna, Madhu *Yantra, The Tantric Symbol Of Cosmic Unity* Thames and Hudson, 1997

Mishra, T N *Impact of Tantra on Religion and Art* D.K. Printworld 1997

Mookerjee, Ajit *Tantra Art* Rupa and Co. 1994

Muir, Charles & Caroline *Tantra, The Art of Conscious Loving* Mercury House Inc. 1989

Odier, Daniel *Tantric Quest, an Encounter With Absolute Love* Inner Traditions, 1997

Osho *The Tantra Experience* Element Books, 1994
Tantric Transformation Element Books, 1994
The Beloved volumes 1&2, Rebel Publishing 1999, 2002
The Book of Secrets St Martin's Press 1998
Sex Matters St Martin's Press, 2002

Ramsdale, David & Ellen *Sexual Energy Ecstasy* Bantam Books, 1993

Richardson, Diana *The Heart of Tantric Sex* Vega Books, 2003

Vatsyayana, trans. Alain Danielou *The Complete Kama Sutra* Park Street Press, 1994

Health and Healing

Allanach, Jack *Colour Me Healing* Vega Press, 2002

Bays, Brandon *The Journey* Thorsons 1999

Jell, Andreas *Healthy With Tachyon* Lotus Press Shangri-La, 2000

Laskow, Leonard, MD *Healing With Love* Wholeness Press, 1992

Lee, John R, MD *What Your Doctor May Not Tell You About Menopause* Warner Books, 1996

Osho *From Medication to Meditation* C W Daniel, 1994

Pert, Candace B, PhD *Molecules of Emotion* Simon and Schuster, 1999

Upledger, John E *Your Inner Physician and You, Craniosacral Therapy and Somatoemotional Release* North Atlantic Books, 1997

Wagner, David & Cousens, Gabriel, MD *Tachyon Energy: A New Paradigm in Holistic Healing* North Atlantic Books, 1999

Willcox, Bradley, MD, Willcox, Craig, PhD & Suzuki, Makoto, MD *The Okinawa Way; How To Improve Your Health And Longevity Dramatically* Penguin Books 2001

Zinovieff, Kolinka *Essential Health, The Complete Aromatherapy Guide* London Natural Health Press, 1997

Childhood and Adolescence

Mai, Anke (ed) *Walking into Beauty, Honouring the Transition into Womanhood* and *First Moon, Celebrating the Onset of Menstruation* Anke Mai, 2002 ankemai@gn.apc.org

Biddulph, Steve *Raising Boys* Thorsons, 1997
The Secret of Happy Children Thorsons, 1998

Meditation

Chopra, Deepak *The Seven Spiritual Laws of Success* Bantam Press, 1996

Osho *Meditation: The First and Last Freedom* St. Martin's Press, 1996
Hidden Mysteries Rebel Publishing, 1997

Empowering Women, Empowering Men

Al-Rawi, Rosina Fawzia *Belly Dancing* Constable & Robinson, 2001

Biddulph, Steve *Manhood* Hawthorn Press, 2002

Dirie, Waris *Desert Flower* Virago Press, 2001

Schlain, Leonard *The Alphabet vs The Goddess* Viking Press, 1998

The Boston Women's Health Book Collective *Our Bodies, Ourselves, A Book by and for Women, for the New Century* Simon and Schuster, 1998

Environment/Indigenous Wisdom

Ereira, Alan *The Elder Brothers, a lost South American people and their wisdom* Vintage Books 1993

Tompkins, Peter & Bird, Christopher *Secrets of the Soil* Earthpulse Press 1998

Holistic therapies and workshops

The therapists and organizations below are all recommended as being of a high standard by ourselves, or by our friends.
Note: Any courses, workshops, or therapy sessions are undertaken at the reader's sole discretion and risk.

For information on the honey cap birth control method:
Harley Place Screening
27 Harley Place
London W1G 8QF
England
Tel: 00 44 (0)20 7323 2383

Northern California
Tantra Initiation Groups (affiliated with The School of Awakening)
Couples Sessions and Colorpuncture
Vibha Call, devavibha@hotmail.com

Bay Area, California
Colorpuncture & Human Design
Kumud Kabir, Hevans@emicfocus.com

Tachyon Institute For Spirituality and Science
David Wagner Tel: 707 573 58 00
www.schoolofawakening-tachyon.com

Sky Dancing Tantra with Margo Anand
skyoffice@infoasis.com,
http://www.spiritworkschurch.net

Family Constellation
Anand Shanti, anandshanti2002@yahoo.com

Herbal Magic
Consultations and natural herbal remedies
Melren@aol.com

Southern California
Eriksonian Hypnosis
Dr Brian Alman, www.selfhypnosis.com

Boulder, Colorado
Institute for Esogetic Colorpuncture, USA
Manohar Croke, CCP, www.colorpuncture.com,
abhmanohar@earthlink.net

Colorpuncture
Jamie St Clair, jamie@sublime-dezine.com

Sarita and Geho are founders of The School of Awakening, based in the UK, which offers courses in aspects of personal development. To contact the authors, to find out about their Tantra trainings for couples and individuals, and to order their meditation CDs, visit their website or write to them at:

The School of Awakening
PO Box 15, Chumleigh,
Devon EX18 7SR
England
Tel: 00 44 (0)1769 581232
www.schoolofawakening.com
info@schoolofawakening.com

Index

Authors' acknowledgements

Our Journey in creating this book has been helped by the following people, to whom we would like to offer our grateful acknowledgements.
The staff of Gaia Books, particularly Joss Pearson, director, Lucy Guenot, designer, Katherine Pate, editor, Steve Teague, photographer, and Jo Godfrey Wood, who initiated the project.
Simon and Schuster who made this book possible with their enthusiastic participation in the publishing of it.
Our amazing models who graciously offered their beauty and charm to these pages, Gitika & Steve, Jivan & Agyana, Anne & Champaka, Pemba & Devi, Niten & Sharona, Al & Kay and Jake.
Our students, whose loving appreciation of our work and whose questions and comments have inspired us to write this book.
Our students, and friends, who have through their interviews and quotes enlivened the text: Jivan and Agyana, Les and Sally, Valerie and Vernon, Tim and Lindy, Kamla and Andrew, Mita and Ajay, Michael, Anne-France, Rachel, Charaka, Archan. With a special thanks to Divyam and Keerti who also helped with research, and special thanks and appreciation also to Al and Kay, who have offered research and inspiration in so many ways. Jake and Rob, thank you so much for giving us quotes to use in the section on childhood. You guys are super! And also to those who gave us quotes on their experience of orgasm, who remain anonymous.
Our lovers; each one of you has given a priceless treasure through your presence in our lives. Each one of you has contributed to this book by enriching our experience of sex and relating on all levels.
Helena Vistara, who helped enormously with the chapter on childhood with her valuable expertise.
Anke Mai, who has offered valuable research for the chapter on adolescence.
Margot Anand, renowned pioneer in the development of Western Tantra, who has prepared the ground for a Tantra renaissance. We are honored that she has endorsed this book.
Naturopath Peter Mandel, whose tremendous insights into healing have benefited us and thousands of others. We have used two of his maps on how human energy functions, in chapter 3.
Glynn Braddy, who has helped with research on men's cycles, and who has also supported the renewal of our health with his alchemical wisdom.
David Wagner, teacher and friend, whose contribution to our wellbeing and to the world is a great blessing. We are ever grateful for his marvellous invention and insights, some of which we have written about.
Korogisan, Zen and Ito-Thermie Master, for his inspiration into the heart of meditation and healing.
Osho, our spiritual master, whose presence is a continuous reminder of our unlimited potential. This book owes its existence to the profound understanding of Tantra offered to us by Osho.
Osho International, for permission to print excerpts from some published and some unpublished works by Osho, from their website: www.osho.com
Ravi, who has composed wonderful music for the Chakra Dance Meditation CD, in time for simultaneous publication with this book.
Supragya and Prasthano, a lovely Tantric couple who also happen to be our office managers. We are so lucky to have them supporting our work in innumerable ways, with so much love and dedication. They are certainly angels in disguise.

Publisher's acknowledgements

Gaia Books would like to thank Deborah Pate for research, Christine Haseler for acting as medical consultant, and Lynn Bresler for the index.
All photography by Steve Teague except pp. 5, 8, 11, Shivananda; pp. 65, 185 Samarpan; pp. 84, 148, 151 Jan Jacobsen; pp.134 , 136, 137 Patrick Leclerc.